Praise for Quiet Mind Quite Body

"*Quiet Mind Quiet Body* is an extraordinary book. The author guides us gently towards an understanding of our true nature that allows us not to just recover from pain but to actually heal. By sharing with us the Three Principles of Mind, Consciousness, and Thought, the author invites us to an understanding that brings harmony between our mind and body. We are guided to realise the happiness, joy and well-being that exists in all of us, and thereby, we are given the potential to transcend pain. If you want to heal your pain and regain your natural peace of mind, well-being and joy, this book is a must-read."

Mark Howard, PhD

Psychologist
Three Principles Institute

ෂාශ

"Through her personal and professional experiences, Julie brings to life the biopsychospiritual understanding of pain. *Quiet Mind Quiet Body* is a gift for anyone experiencing chronic pain, as well as those health professionals supporting people who have pain. This book has the potential to change the course of well-being throughout the world!"

Ellen Friedman, MA, PT (ret.)

Soul-Centered Professional Coach,
Three Principles Practitioner

"This book is a blessing for all those who suffer with pain as well as those who care for them. Julie writes from a wealth of experience, both personal and professional, but she also writes from the heart. This is not just another 'pain management' book. It is a book that will expand your understanding of pain, opening your heart and mind to self-healing possibilities that may never have occurred to you before. If you're looking for a more loving, gentle and compassionate approach to pain relief, I can highly recommend this book."

Ian Watson

Wellbeing Educator at The Insight Space

ಲ೦ಣ

"*Quiet Mind Quiet Body* opened new ways for me to understand and promote healing of chronic pain – mine and those of my clients. Both hopeful and insightful, this book is a must-read for healthcare professionals and their hurting patients – really, for everyone who walks around in a body! Julie McCammon's heartfelt expertise and wisdom shine."

Linda Sandel Pettit, Ed.D.

Author and Influencer
at the Intersection of Spirituality and Psychology

"Julie shares an understanding that goes beyond the traditional physical explanations of pain. What makes this compelling is that Julie doesn't speak from theories or concepts; this is her lived experience resolving many chronic pain conditions with what can appear to be miraculous results. This book isn't about raising your hopes – it's about deepening your understanding so that you realise your access to such results."

Dominic Scaffidi

Master Certified Coach

❧☙

"Julie McCammon has written a brilliant book. She combines her years of training in various modalities to create a groundbreaking book on pain and a new way to approach it. Bravo!"

Ankush Jain

Coach and Author of
Sweet Sharing: Rediscovering the REAL You

"Julie McCammon is a physiotherapist and expert-level Myofascial Release therapist who wrote this in her excellent book, *Quiet Mind Quiet Body*: "Your soul will meet you in the stillness."

I had the opportunity to treat Julie when she was in the midst of very deep pain. She is a very brave woman. She is articulate and has reached into the very depths of the human experience. I highly recommend her book."

John F. Barnes, PT

Myofascial Release Treatment Centers & Seminars

ಬಿಲ್ಲ

"Chronic pain is a blight on the lives of millions, and healing often requires a journey of body, mind, and spirit. While an understanding of the neurological mechanisms of pain has brought relief to many, most of that work has overlooked the spiritual dimension, leaving countless individuals still searching for true relief. Julie McCammon's work bridges this gap, illuminating a new way forward for those seeking lasting peace."

Jamie Smart

Sunday Times Bestselling Author

"Through personal experience and deep study, Julie shows us over several chapters the ways that we all have access to that space beyond thought... where the soul waits to guide us to the meaning behind what we are experiencing in our bodies. She encourages us to let go of resistance, to gently breathe and ask for guidance... to let go of the need to control and fix our body, and finally, to trust that we are being pulled towards health and wholeness. We have what it takes to use our hearts and our minds to heal from the inside out."

Carol M. Davis, DPT, EdD, MS, FAPTA

Myofascial Release Physical Therapist
Professor Emerita
Department of Physical Therapy
University of Miami Miller School of Medicine

Quiet Mind
Quiet Body

Julie McCammon

First published in Great Britain in 2025
by Whispering Body Press

© Copyright Julie McCammon 2025

The moral right of Julie McCammon to be identified as the author of this work has been asserted in accordance with the Copyright, Designs and Patents Acts 1988.

All rights reserved. No part of this publication may be reproduced, stored in a retrieval system, or transmitted, in any form or by any means without the prior written permission of the publisher, nor be otherwise circulated in any form of binding or cover than that in which it is published and without similar condition being imposed on the subsequent purchaser.

A CIP catalogue record for this book
is available at the British Library.

ISBN (Paperback) 978-1-0682368-0-8
ISBN (eBook) 978-1-0682368-1-5

To my love, Peter.

My greatest cheerleader and my unwavering support.
Your love lifts me, your belief in me never falters,
and your presence is my greatest gift.

With all my love, always.

Contents

Foreword	1
Introduction: The Red Armchair	5
Chapter 1: Quiet Mind Quiet Body	9
Chapter 2: Brain-Body-Soul: Understanding of Pain – Biopsychospiritual Model	15
Chapter 3: Experiencing Pain	23
Chapter 4: How Our Experience is Created	29
Chapter 5: You Can't Sneak a Thought Past the Body	37
Chapter 6: The Feeling is Foolproof	53
Chapter 7: This is the Age of Well-Being	61
Chapter 8: Understanding Pain	71
Chapter 9: Re-Thinking Pain	83
Chapter 10: Words Create Our Reality	97
Chapter 11: Soul's Wisdom	103
Chapter 12: Harnessing the Wisdom of Your Body	115
Chapter 13: Our Guide Inside	125
Chapter 14: Mercy and Tenderness Heals	131
Appendices	
Journaling Questions	137
Glossary of Terms	141
Further Reading and Resources	145
With Deepest Gratitude	155
About the Author	159

Foreword

IN READING *QUIET MIND QUIET BODY*, you are giving yourself a profound gift – one that awakens fresh hope, deepens self-understanding, and offers the possibility of true healing. This book has the power to transform not only your relationship with pain but also your relationship with yourself and others.

Throughout my 50+ years as a physician, more than 40 years as a psychiatrist, and nearly 15 years as a mentor and coach, I have encountered the pervasive and relentless impact of chronic pain. It is an ever-present spectre in the lives of so many, often dictating the terms of their daily existence.

A simple search for "chronic stress" and "chronic pain" in the U.S. National Library of Medicine yields over 300,000 articles – evidence of just how deeply these conditions affect our world. In 2016, a landmark study spanning 195 countries was published in the prestigious journal *Nature*. The findings highlighted significant disparities in mortality rates based on socioeconomic status. Yet, when it came to disability-related diagnoses, neck and back pain consistently ranked among the top three across all nations. Chronic pain knows no boundaries; it is a universal human challenge.

If you or a loved one has endured years of seeking relief from persistent pain without success, I urge you to approach this book with an open heart and mind. Read it once, then read it again. The insights within these pages are revolutionary and evolutionary – challenging long-held unconscious beliefs about pain and healing.

The author speaks from a place of deep wisdom, drawn from personal experience, scientific research, and a lifelong commitment to the healing professions. The truth she points to is not merely intellectual; it resonates at the deepest level of consciousness, awakening the formless spiritual wisdom within. As you read, realisations will emerge – effortlessly yet profoundly – allowing you to release what no longer serves you while retaining the genuine gold of lived experience.

On your second reading, you will see with new eyes and hear with new ears. What once seemed complex or overwhelming will become clear and simple. The spiritual nature of life – so often hidden beneath layers of misunderstanding – will come into sharper focus, offering peace where there was once struggle.

I wholeheartedly recommend this book to every human being, for who among us has not faced moments of emotional or physical pain that challenged our understanding? To my fellow physicians, nurses, psychologists, and all in the healing professions, I especially commend this work. In rediscovering the love and wisdom at the core of our being, we can more confidently and compassionately guide those who seek our help on their journey home to peace.

Simply stated, *Quiet Mind Quiet Body* carries a profound message that has the potential to transform the world by elevating the state of being of all who embrace it.

William F. Pettit, M.D.

Board-certified psychiatrist, co-owner of 3 Principles Intervention LLC, and international educator on the Three Universal Principles of Mind, Consciousness, and Thought.

Introduction

The Red Armchair

I SIT IN THE WELL-WORN red armchair with my two cocker spaniels curled up beside me. Each day, my morning ritual involves reading and quiet, space for the flow of creativity as I voyage into the heart of mystery.

Today, I reflect on how my life has been a magical journey, a path of the alchemist. I have taken each experience, good and bad, and turned the ordinary into gold, making medicine from my pain.

This magic is available to us all.

My purpose is to bring hope and healing through the power of this creation.

I see the play of the universe and soul that has brought me to my purpose – writing *Quiet Mind Quiet Body*.

Despite struggling academically, I worked hard and gained an Honours Degree in Physiotherapy, graduating in 1990. Then, in 2015, after struggling with my health for over 15 years, I stumbled upon Myofascial Release Therapy (MFR), which brought so much freedom to my body and mind. I spent the next five years travelling back and forth to America from Ireland to become an expert-level John F. Barnes Myofascial Release Therapist. I attended training seminars, and I also deepened my journey of healing and expansion by receiving treatment during this time.

I have always followed a path of curiosity, and this path brought me to an understanding called the Three Principles in 2022. Following other prompts, I signed up to work with Dr Linda Sandel Petitt, a personal consultant whose work is steeped in this understanding of how the mind works. Little did I know the journey that decision would take me on, a journey of healing from the inside out. Linda is my mentor and a truly amazing intuitive guide. She is one of the wisest and most beautiful souls I have ever had the pleasure of meeting.

I have had the privilege of studying both the body and the mind and how the bodymind contributes to our experience of life. In 2024, inspired to help others in a way that combines these understandings, I completed a six-month Three Principle Practitioner Training programme at Regent's University London, with the equally amazing Ian Watson.

Introduction: The Red Armchair

I am being called to study my passion in the deepest way available as I continue to bump up against my growth edges.

Our experience is constantly attempting to communicate with us, but we human beings forget how to listen. My path has been filled with mystery, and many times I've ignored the guidance, but somehow, I've managed eventually to hear the nudges. Looking back, I followed the breadcrumbs that life has offered me, from Physiotherapy to Myofascial Release Therapy to Three Principles to Bodymind Coaching. I have trusted the invisible golden thread that is woven into the unique pattern that is my life. It has brought me precisely to where I am today, sitting in my red armchair, filled with purpose and passion for writing this book as an act of service to anyone who is struggling with persistent pain or feeling overwhelmed by anxious thinking.

Pain, whether emotional or physical, can be seen as an irritant, but through incremental insight, it can become a treasure – the grit that creates a pearl. My pain inspires me to share what I have learned along the way.

My life has shown me that where I stumble, there lies my treasure. Each step of the path allows me to gather seeds, enabling me to develop my own way of sharing and evolving.

As I step into the unknown, I will bring the totality of my experience and share it with you in the pages of this book.

We are all alchemists.

We all have a deep and timeless wisdom that arises from the within.

We are all making medicine with our thoughts and intentions.

I intend to create opportunities for healing in the world by combining science and wisdom to unlock the mystery of the Mind so that you, dear reader, can find freedom from pain and suffering.

Julie McCammon

May 2025

Chapter 1

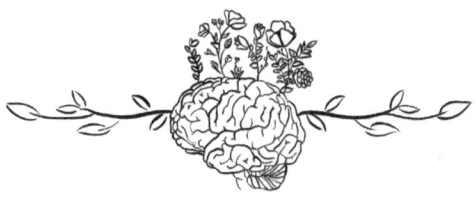

Quiet Mind Quiet Body

QUIET MIND QUIET BODY has the potential to help you see and experience life in a completely new way.

In these pages, I will shine a light, like morning sunlight on a spider's web, to show you the threads of an invisible web which connects body and mind. I hope that you gain your own personal insights as you read these pages. Each insight will take up residence in your bones and cause a deep, abiding, embodied shift in your consciousness. May these words carry the potential for quiet transformation.

My story of persistent pain started in 1999 when, following viral meningitis, I developed post-viral fatigue. Choosing to ignore my body's whispers for years, this then developed into chronic fatigue and eventually fibromyalgia-like symptoms. My condition progressed over 15 years – years of pushing through and ignoring my body's wisdom, which brought me to a breaking point. From there, I discovered a new healing modality called Myofascial Release Therapy. This is the story of my first book, *Finding Mystery Within*.

I also suffered what began as an acute episode of lower back pain and left leg sciatica in 2018, which was one of the most painful experiences of my life and lasted over 18 weeks. Yet again, I fell into a chronic pain cycle fuelled by fear. If I – a physiotherapist – couldn't fix my own back, how could I fix my patients? Would I need surgery? For years, I had told patients to avoid surgery like the plague! I realised that by giving life and attention to these thoughts, I had created a cycle of overtreating and not listening to my body. I was attached to the outcome and could not let go.

It wasn't until I stumbled across the metaphor of the Three Principles in 2020 that I truly began to understand why the pain persisted for so long and why it left overnight following an insight I had after simply reading a poem. I don't remember anything about the poem – who it was by or what is contained – but it enabled me to escape the storm in my mind and begin detaching from the outcome. The Principles point towards understanding the nature of the mind and how it works, how our experience is only and always created from the inside out, and how it is impossible for us to be broken as we have everything we need inside ourselves.

I hope the information in this book will unlock the mystery of the mind and bring freedom from suffering, as it has done for me and many others.

I began writing a journal when I was 12. I am still writing because I am compelled to find meaning in my experience. I am always observing, noting, comparing, and articulating.

Finding Mystery Within was my first attempt at writing a book. It was born during the COVID-19 lockdown out of a desire to understand and document the nature of my healing journey. Since then, it has become increasingly clear that the way to bring healing is by discovering a connection between body and mind.

The power of Thought is the bridge between the two. I believe the Three Principles' understanding provides a meeting place for the body and mind, allowing them to walk through life together as a 'bodymind'.

For the first 45 years, I journeyed solely in my head; I was only aware of, conscious of, what was going on in my brain – in my thinking. My mind was 100% in the driver's seat. Despite training as a physiotherapist, working with the body, my training was all about the brain, intellect, and science.

As mentioned, in 2015, I came across Myofascial Release Therapy, which blew my mind wide open. My focus became more on the body, and when I dropped out of my head and into my body, a whole new world opened up.

Thanks to my husband, Peter, I was introduced to the metaphor of the Three Universal Principles: Mind, Consciousness, and Thought. These Principles point to the spiritual truth of what we as human beings are and the gifts we have each been given to create our experience, one thought at a time from the inside out. My continued curiosity has led me to write this book.

The stories on these pages will resonate with you, because we are all subject to illness, pain and ageing. We may have spent months or years in despair that the answer is forever out of reach, having already tried everything to soothe or relieve our pain.

Some of us find ourselves, not by choice, inhabiting a state of persistent pain. If we are so inclined, we can innocently slip into a heightened state of awareness. If you or someone you know is yearning to find a way out of the cycle of persistent pain, please keep reading.

Whether you long for a life where you can play with your kids unhindered, hunger for a day filled with happy memories instead of pain-limiting ones, dream of scaling a mountain or even a small hill, or long to ease the pain, these are all manifestations of the same ache: to live a life free from suffering and to feel at home in your own body. We are all reaching for something.

I will explain how you can transform the way you experience pain and help you understand the relationship between the body and mind.

Quiet Mind Quiet Body has the potential to transform pain into beauty.

Key Takeaways

◊ **Connecting Body and Mind:** A quiet mind leads to a quiet body.

◊ **My Personal Healing Journey:** Years of ignoring signals until I had an insight.

◊ **Transformation Through New Insights:** Shifting the focus from intellect to the body's wisdom via the Three Principles.

◊ **Invitation to Embrace Change:** Inviting you to embark of your own journey of transforming pain into beauty.

Chapter 2

Brain-Body-Soul: Understanding of Pain – Biopsychospiritual Model

IT'S HARD TO BELIEVE THERE was a time before the 1600s when pain was seen as a punishment or a penance from God to atone for immoral acts. We've come a long way since then!

In 1644, French philosopher René Descartes bravely proposed that pain originated not in the angelic realms but in the brain (*Treatise of Man/Traite de l'Homme*). Pain became a subject of scientific interest, and Descartes's proposal laid the groundwork for the evolution of pain theories.

Reflecting on my university years as a physiotherapy student, I was taught the prevailing belief that all pain was a direct result of injury, transmitted from the injury site to the brain. Emphasis was placed on a strictly biomedical model, with the body and brain as separate entities. Little did I know then that this understanding would undergo a significant transformation.

In the 1960s, Melzack and Wall introduced the now prevalent Pain Gate Theory, which suggested that the intensity of a painful stimulus does not solely determine the perception of pain; it is also influenced by other factors such as emotional state, attention, and expectations. In the 1970s, other theories and research also pointed towards the importance of psychological and social factors in the experience of pain. Hence, a biopsychosocial model developed, and a shift towards the mind as opposed to the brain began. Let me clarify the difference here. The brain is like a computer; it's the anatomical, physical structure that can be held during an anatomy dissection, while the Mind is spiritual and cannot be held or contained. The Mind is formless.

This points beyond these current understandings in the direction of a *biopsychospiritual* understanding of pain. This newest model brings the body, mind, and soul into the frame in a desire to fully understand pain, often referred to as "mind-body" pain.

Timeline

1900s   Biomedical Model – Brain/ Body Divide

1970s   Biopsychosocial Model

2000s   Mindbody Pain/Psychogenic Pain

2025   Biopsychospiritual Model

The biopsychospiritual model is a significant development! It explains the unexplainable.

Understanding the mind can also help us understand how pain can exist without a structural cause. It provides hope for the patients who have been told there is no tissue injury found or that they are making their pain up, that it's all in their head.

I learned about the biomedical model when I earned my degree in Physiotherapy in the 1980s. In the last 20 years, through my health issues, I gradually became aware of the psychological factors that were influencing my experience of pain. Sad to say, I still viewed the body and mind as separate until around eight years ago when I stumbled upon Myofascial Release Therapy, which very much revealed to me that the body and mind cannot be separated.

During my Myofascial Release training, I experienced deep bracing and tension in my body that I wasn't even aware of because I spent most of my time in my head, totally ignoring my body. The tension and bracing had become so habitual, it was not in my awareness until I learned how to give and receive this deeply healing treatment. I then became incrementally aware of the impact our thinking has on our bodies. Up to this point, I had somehow managed to live life almost exclusively from the neck up, but now I could not ignore that I am mind and body in one. We are, after all, spiritual beings having a human experience.

> *"We are not human beings having a spiritual experience. We are spiritual beings having a human experience."*
>
> Teilhard de Chardin (1881-1955)
> French priest, philosopher and scientist

When I came across the Three Principles in 2020 (also known as the Inside Out Understanding), I began to see that we all have access to wisdom beyond the intellect. In 1973, a welder from Scotland named Sydney Banks stepped forward to suggest there were Three Principles, three invisible powers, that explained how we create our personal reality from the inside out. The Three Principles are the fundamental nature of human experience through Mind, Consciousness, and Thought. I will expand on this in Chapter 4, but for now, this understanding reveals that our feelings come from 'thought' in the moment, not external circumstances, offering deep insight into well-being, resilience, and the innate health within us all. It made so much sense to me that all the thoughts we believe are what create our experience of life. If we give life to anxious thoughts, we will feel anxious; if we give life to sad thoughts, we will feel sad.

Understanding the Three Principles could open up a new way of understanding pain.

Pain is a multifaceted phenomenon involving not only the physical body but also the psychological and spiritual aspects of human experience.

Pain is not simply a signal that something is wrong in the body but rather a protective response generated by our mind's response to perceived threats. In other words, thoughts and thinking can contribute to the experience of pain.

My goal is to challenge traditional pain models and help shift the focus of pain management to a more insightful, hopeful approach that considers the Mind's role and its contribution to pain. By unlocking the mystery of the mind, we find freedom from suffering.

What is a Biopsychospiritual Model?

The biological aspect of the model focuses on the body and brain, the physiological processes that contribute to health and illness.

The psychological aspect of the model recognises the role of the mental and emotional states, attitudes, beliefs and behaviours in influencing health outcomes.

The spiritual aspect of the model points us towards the fact that there is something beyond us. Lisa Miller, in her book *The Awakened Brain,* states that "spirituality is a consciousness for which *all* of our brains are wired". Sydney Banks's Three Principles point us towards the spiritual wisdom that lies within the consciousness of *all* human beings. We will consider the inside-out nature of our experience and how we use the gift of Thought to create our experience. Including the spiritual in our understanding of pain offers hope that we are never broken and lack nothing.

Imagine a man in his forties who suffers an acute episode of lower back pain. He works as a manual labourer on a building site. He has three small children, and his wife is a stay-at-home mum. He starts to panic, thinking about how his family will survive if he cannot return to his job. He innocently gets caught up in a cycle of fearful thinking. He becomes irritable with his wife and kids, beating himself up for failure and inability to provide for his family.

As you continue to read, you will understand how this fear cycle becomes a pain cycle, causing the patient to experience chronic pain (pain that lasts longer than three months after injury). The pain is real, but when you are stuck in a fear cycle, you will experience pain at a much lower level of stimulus.

Life is not only a science; it is a creation and an art!

This biopsychospiritual model looks at how a person's thoughts, emotions, and actions affect their pain. It encourages individuals to take an active role in their recovery rather than relying only on external treatments such as medication or surgery, which often fail to help people with chronic pain.

Key Takeaways

◊ **Evolution of Pain Theories:** From Divine Punishment, to the current biopsychospiritual model integrating body, mind, and soul.

◊ **Biopsychospiritual Model:** Recognising pain as a multifaceted experience with thoughts, emotions, and beliefs influencing physical health, highlighting the interconnectedness of mind and body.

◊ **The Mind's Role in Pain:** Understanding the "inside-out" nature of experience – how thoughts shape feelings – helps break fear-pain cycles and fosters healing.

◊ **Empowerment and Hope:** A shift from external treatments to personal responsibility for recovery, providing hope and advocating for holistic, patient-centred care.

Chapter 3

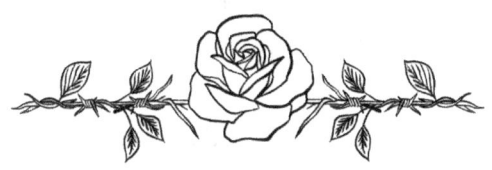

Experiencing Pain

QUIET MIND QUIET BODY focuses on transforming your experience of pain and enhancing your understanding of how the body and mind function. Approaching this book with a sense of wonder will provide you with insights and realisations that facilitate the transformation of pain into beauty.

The essence of the book revolves around responding to pain: acknowledging it and striving to transform it into healing and growth that nourishes the soul. If this seems improbable, even impossible, please bear with me! My life and work have led me to this truth.

Each time you experience pain, it changes you slightly. You either become imprisoned by it or something shifts, allowing you to discover more freedom than you ever believed possible. Pain happens repeatedly, and we can view it as a great tragedy or something wise trying to capture our attention. Pain is unavoidable, and we tend to think that suffering with it is inevitable. This book intends to help you understand where suffering comes from. Then, you will have the option to stop it at its source.

Explaining the Unexplainable

Understanding pain can be like explaining the unexplainable, but I promise to keep it simple.

The most significant misunderstanding about pain is that all pain is caused by a structural issue. *This is a myth that needs to be busted!*

Doctors working in frontline situations, such as GP surgeries or Emergency Rooms, can see that the current biomedical model does not fully explain chronic pain. They know this because patients with long-standing pain keep returning for help. This current biomedical model for chronic pain is outdated. It puts patients with chronic pain into one of three categories.

1. There must be a structural issue causing the pain, and when doctors cannot find a structural problem with scans or X-rays, chronic pain patients are moved into category two or three.

2. No structural cause can be found in the investigation, so the patient's pain is not real – devastating news for patients, causing even more stress and anxiety.

3. There is evidence on a scan, so the doctor says, "Ah, this is the cause of your pain; we can operate to fix it." Unfortunately, this abnormality is not the cause of their pain, so the surgery fails, and the cycle continues. Research shows 'abnormalities' exist in high occurrences in pain-free people, so it is not the cause of their chronic pain in the first place. Yes, you read that correctly; the same structural issue that appears to cause pain for one person may not cause pain in another!! So next time your scan results show wear and tear or 'damage' – consider that this may not necessarily be the cause of your pain.

Since the current biomedical model fails these patients, it may be time to consider a different approach.

The outdated biomedical model, that unfortunately many healthcare professionals still work with, suggests that structural pain is real and non-structural pain is not. All too often, when a structural issue, such as an acute injury, inflammation, or nerve damage, isn't found, patients may feel they are being told their symptoms are all in their heads. I want to reassure you that **all pain is real!**

Conditions such as fibromyalgia, non-specific lower back pain, chronic migraines, tension headaches, chronic temporomandibular pain disorders or chronic neck/back pain fall into this nociplastic pain/chronic pain/persistent pain category. The list is endless.

> Nociplastic pain is a chronic condition arising from altered pain-related pathways in the central nervous system and periphery. Often, it has no clinical reasoning or mechanism of action. It is distinct in that the pain migrates, described by patients as diffuse, and they often can't locate the pain.

Pain is a Marker of Protection

In recent years, several experts, such as Dr John E. Sarno, Dr Howard Schubiner, and Dr Lorimer Moseley, have bravely started to point in another direction. They see the need to shift from the older biomedical model to something new. Their huge bodies of research and exploration (see *Further Reading and Resources*) into a new understanding of why pain persists long after the body has healed the initial injury, are bringing hope to chronic pain sufferers.

Experts are beginning to point towards pain being a marker of *protection* and not always a marker of *detection or abnormality*. Our nervous system is simply trying to protect us by producing pain, which prevents movement and allows injured tissues to heal by avoiding mechanical forces from exceeding the injured tissue's strength in its injured state. When we give our fearful and anxious thoughts about our health too much attention, we give them all the power, triggering an already oversensitive nervous system, perpetuating our pain well beyond the time it takes our body to heal the initial injury.

The role of our personal mind in innocently perpetuating/causing chronic pain is the key that has been overlooked for too long. Consider this: What if pain or symptoms are not only markers of pathology but rather our body's way of attempting to guide us towards a state of greater wholeness? Could pain be guiding us away from our thoughts and into our lives, into the silence of 'now' where wisdom lives? Could symptoms be a protective mechanism, your deeper wisdom stopping you from continuing on a path that could destroy you?

As long as we continue to think 'pain' is a problem and we reach for a quick fix, we are unlikely to consider that our body might be trying to get our attention.

Key Takeaways

◊ **Transforming Pain:** Pain can be a guide towards healing and growth so we need to view pain as a call to greater awareness and freedom.

◊ **Rethinking Pain's Cause:** Critiquing an outdated biomedical model of chronic pain that points to structural causes alone, highlighting the need for acceptance of non-structural causes of chronic pain.

◊ **Pain as Protection:** Reframing pain as a protective response by the nervous system, emphasising the role of fear and anxious thoughts in perpetuating chronic pain.

◊ **Holistic Perspective:** Advocating a new approach to pain, suggesting the body's wisdom guides us to better choices and greater wholeness.

Chapter 4

How Our Experience is Created

BEFORE WE EXAMINE THE neuroscience behind pain in greater depth and understand fully how the body works, we must understand how the mind works and how human experience is created. After years of trying to understand pain by separating the body and the mind, we have realised it is an interwoven system.

In her book *Molecules of Emotion*, Dr Candace Pert states, *"Most psychologists treat the mind as disembodied, a phenomenon with little or no connection to the physical body. Conversely, physicians treat the body with no regard to the mind or the emotions. But the body and mind are not separate, and we cannot treat one without the other. My research has shown me that the body can and must be healed through the mind, and the mind can and must be healed through the body."*

You might have heard it called the 'bodymind' or the 'mindbody'; which one doesn't matter. What matters is that we understand that we are thinking creatures and use our minds to create our experience of life from the inside out, which intimately affects our bodies.

It's a profound truth that we shape our experiences of any situation or circumstance through our thoughts. Consider two individuals in the same scenario who don't perceive it in the same way. For instance, while waiting in line at the grocery store, one person feels annoyed by the customer in front and the chatty cashier taking forever to complete their transaction. Meanwhile, another relishes the opportunity to pause amid a hectic day. The only differentiating factor is each individual's 'Thoughts'.

Our feelings do not result from external events but always from our thoughts about them. Therefore, we can only feel what we think.

As we each create our personal reality from within our mind, this helps us understand why we often experience the same outside circumstances differently than someone else. Not everyone has road rage, thank goodness. Believe it or not, 'Thought' creates our responses to the weather or traffic. This hit me one day when I was walking the dogs around our local lake. It was a dull, grey day, and as I walked, I thought, "What a depressing day." One minute later, as I turned the corner and headed towards the waterfall, I met a gentleman walking towards me; we nodded and said hello as we passed, and he then commented, "Isn't it a lovely day?" I almost laughed as I heard myself agree, "Yes, it is indeed!"

We live in a world where we each create separate realities based on our unique collection of personal thoughts, beliefs, attitudes, and our states of mind. We all have different thoughts depending on our past experiences, beliefs, and prejudices based on our personal history. When we realise our feelings and experiences are not coming from "out there" but from our thoughts in the moment, we find the freedom to react or not to react to our thinking.

It has been suggested that we have anywhere between 6,000 to 60,000 thoughts daily; 90% of which are repetitive. Most of these thoughts are rooted in our memories, but occasionally, a novel, innovative thought slips through when our minds settle. When we find ourselves in the space of a quiet mind, we are in the realm of pure potential, the birthplace of inventions. Sydney Banks refers to how everyone has spiritual wisdom before the intellect; it lies in the consciousness of all human beings! In this space, we are awakened to new ways of living, behaving, problem-solving, and experiencing joy.

We've all found ourselves in situations where we struggle with a problem, unable to find a solution because our thoughts are on repeat, leading us down the same dead end. Suddenly, in the shower or while walking the dogs, where our minds are a little quieter, the solution pops into our minds as clear as day. Where did that fresh new thought come from?

There is a spiritual space beyond thought where well-being and clarity reside. **Every** human being has access to this space.

We each have a formless spiritual wisdom, a place of love inside, that can give us what we yearn for – a life free from suffering. The noise of our thoughts, the voice inside our heads, obscures our innate health and well-being. Better answers lie within us. Throughout history, sages have referred to this place in various ways – the Mind; God; the still, small voice. This space has the potential to bring you happiness, and is somewhere that you feel fully alive in a beautiful body that is exquisitely designed.

When we transcend pain, even momentarily, we find 'ourselves' fading away and feel connected to something bigger, having a profound experience of the oneness of life.

Sydney Banks's Three Principles were Mind, Consciousness, and Thought. These Principles are metaphors he used to explain his direct experience of the Divine. This understanding has helped me better understand the exquisite connection and interplay between the body, mind, and soul. Here is my understanding of them:

> **Mind** is formless energy, the divine intelligence behind all of life. It is present in everything and everyone. We see it in nature when a flower turns towards the sun; we see it in our bodies when a cut begins to close over and heal, or when our heart knows when to take its next beat. We are all Mind and are all guided in life, whether we realise it or not. We are not separate from that which is behind life.

Consciousness is a miraculous gift we have been given in order to experience life. We need it to be aware of everything and anything. Life would be very different if we did not have this gift. It would be like living under a general anaesthetic. We would breathe, but not see, hear, smell, taste, or feel anything. It would not be much of a life and we would miss out on so, so much!

Thought is another incredible gift that comes from the formless and helps us create our own experiences in life. A thought takes no effort; it simply happens. We have no control over which thoughts pop into our minds, but it's important to know that we don't have to engage with every thought. If we grab hold of every thought that enters our minds and believe it to be true, it will only cause suffering (except for happy thoughts).

We can use our thinking to hurt or to heal (thinking is the act of thinking about our thoughts.) When we understand that a feeling accompanies every thought, we can follow the thoughts that give us a nicer feeling, such as joy, peace, and love, rather than dwelling on thoughts that result in tension, anxiety, or fear. We know that what we experience directly results from the thoughts and thinking we entertain.

These Three Principles are three divine gifts we are given to help us navigate this experience and spiritual journey we call life.

We are the thinkers and creators of our experience, with no exceptions. We use the power of Thought to create the reality we see, and what we experience depends on whether those thoughts are positive or negative, conscious or unconscious, actual or illusionary. Our perception of reality seems very true to us. We will feel what we think, and our feelings are real.

The good news is that we can shift what we are experiencing when we SEE that our thoughts are creating our experience. So, it's not about trying to control or change our thinking from negative to positive as this only offers a temporary solution. It is simply about recognising the power that our thoughts have over us and choosing to let a particular thought pass rather than believing it or grabbing hold of it. We are only ever one thought away from an entirely new experience!

> *"You are one thought away from happiness,*
> *one thought away from sadness.*
> *The secret lies in thought"*
>
> Sydney Banks

This understanding points us back to the now, to common sense and wisdom that lie within our own consciousness. It allows us to weather storms, avoid obstacles, and adjust our course when we get lost and caught up in our thinking. If we do not believe everything we think, there is space for us to hear and respond to the wisdom that is within us, and this alone helps us avoid needless suffering.

Psychological stress is not linked to circumstances and events outside the individual but to their thinking in the moment. So, rather than getting lost and searching outside ourselves to change our feelings, we should turn inward and see how our life experience is created. Then, we will rediscover our inner strength and our innate capacity for health and well-being.

Key Takeaways

◊ **Interconnected Mind-Body System:** The inseparable link between the mind and body, with thoughts playing a central role in how we perceive and respond to pain.

◊ **Creation of Experience:** Our experiences are created from thoughts, and feelings are always a direct result of thoughts, not circumstances.

◊ **Accessing Inner Clarity:** The quieter mind accesses wisdom, clarity, and innovative solutions, highlighting the potential of focusing on positive, healing thoughts.

◊ **Three Principles of Experience:** Understanding the Three Principles of Mind (divine intelligence), Consciousness (awareness), and Thought (the power to create reality) help us reduce suffering and find our innate well-being.

Chapter 5

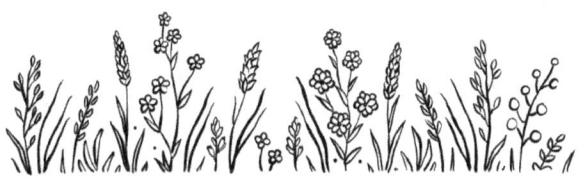

You Can't Sneak a Thought Past the Body

My Story

I TWISTED TO GET OUT of the car, and my lower back tightened. It had been a long day treating clients in my physiotherapy clinic; I was tired but satisfied with the day's work. My back didn't hurt, but it felt tense and stiff. The sensation appeared out of nowhere.

I went to bed, thinking all would be fine after a night's rest, but the next morning I still felt stiff. I was due to attend a yin yoga class, and I decided to go ahead, thinking the gentle stretching would help. I had just finished my breakfast at the kitchen table, and I leaned forward to tie my shoelaces; I was gripped by the most intense pain I had felt since childbirth. It was so severe that I screamed out for help. My husband ran into the kitchen to offer his support. I was stuck; I couldn't straighten up; I even found breathing difficult, and the room began to spin.

I put all my weight on my arms on the kitchen table as I attempted to stand, but the pain took my breath away each time I tried. The tears began to spill down my face, and I felt trapped in my chair, unable to move.

After many attempts, I eventually got onto all fours on the tiled floor. On my hands and knees, I crawled to the other end of the kitchen, where the floor was carpeted. I got myself onto my back and did very gentle, appeasing exercises – exercises I had taught countless patients with lumbar spine issues to do.

I might have laughed if I wasn't in such severe pain. There I was, a physiotherapist who specialised in treating lower back pain and neck pain, needing to practice what I had preached for over 20 years.

I spent the next 18 weeks on the floor. I crawled until I was able to use crutches to walk. The pain went from my back into my left leg. The sciatica pain was exhausting and unrelenting. Every single thing I attempted to do triggered my pain.

I went for a scan after about four weeks, when I could eventually manage the car journey. The results showed that I had a tear in the annular wall of my L4/L5 disc on the left side, causing pressure on the nerve root as it exited the spine at that level.

I commenced physiotherapy treatment twice a week and did everything I knew to do at home in between. I was determined to fix this problem.

My mind was swirling with thoughts.

"How could I fix my patients if I couldn't fix my own back?" and "Will I need surgery?" (despite advising my patients for years to avoid surgery like the plague!)

I became obsessed. Only looking back now can I see how I was overtreating myself – I was catastrophising!

After almost 18 weeks of pain, I was sure my disc would have healed itself. I knew I was heading into a 'chronic pain' cycle that would be virtually impossible to get out of. I was gripped by fear!

It was a Sunday evening; I had just read a poem on Facebook. I don't remember the poem or what it said, but my racing mind quieted down. I told myself, "You know what, Julie, you are going to be OK; even if you need surgery, you will be OK!" Then, within my mind, I heard, "You need to detach from the outcome." I had often heard one of my teachers, John F. Barnes, speak those words.

I went to sleep feeling peaceful despite my persistent pain. The following day, I woke up with virtually no pain. I had somehow turned a corner by letting go of my commentary, the struggling, the resisting, the self-pity, the worry, and the fear.

Until that day, I had been resisting what was, with every fibre of my being. My personal experience is what we resist persists! This insight allowed me to see the mind-body connection between my stressful thinking and my persistent pain.

Something shifted in my understanding of pain. I saw that all pain is not structural; sometimes, it's more psychological and neurological in nature. My mind had become stuck in hypervigilance, worry and stress, causing my body to be held prisoner in a pain loop that was really a fear loop. My invisible thinking told my nervous system that I was not safe, and so it remained in a constant state of fight-or-flight. Catching a glimpse of this allowed me to see that the more I dropped out of my vigilant thinking, the more my body relaxed, and my symptoms abated. In other words, I got out of my head and into my life!

I began to realise the power of my thoughts over my body.

I saw that being comfortable with what is promotes healing. This all happened before I had even heard about the Three Principles, proving that they always exist, whether we know them or not, like the principle of gravity.

Let me explain. I want you to imagine your favourite dessert, or pudding as we call it here in Northern Ireland, on the table before you. If you don't have a sweet tooth, imagine something savoury or salty. Chocolate brownies float my boat, still moist and soft in the middle, served slightly warm with Swedish glaze dairy-free ice cream melting on top.

Imagine you are about to take a bite. The odds are that you can begin to feel saliva pooling inside your mouth. The thought of the food produced a response in your body.

Now, bring to mind something or someone you think makes you angry or upset.

Where do you feel it in your body? You might feel tension in your shoulders, clenching in your jaw, or even a tightness in your stomach. Hear me when I say you can't sneak a thought past your body!!

I invite you to try it now. Give yourself the gift of feeling your thoughts in your body as you bring to mind something that you believe causes you to feel stressed.

Every thought that we give attention to produces a feeling in the body, whether we are conscious of it or not. A feeling of fear cannot happen without a thought of fear. But the feeling often happens so fast that we don't even notice that there was a thought.

The feelings we feel as a result of our thoughts feel so real that they affect us physically. I grew up in Northern Ireland during the 60s and 70s, at the height of The Troubles, a time of conflict when many lost their lives in the daily bombings and shootings. Living in a small border village, it was a regular occurrence to hear of someone we knew who had been shot or to feel the shockwaves of a bomb travel through the town.

We lived above my parents' grocery store, which served both sides of the community, making us a target, and our home was even bombed on one occasion.

For many years after moving away from the village, loud noises often triggered a physical response in my body, causing contractions and bracing while my heart raced. I would have a visceral reaction, physically bending over and crouching for cover, only to discover it was a car backfiring.

Such reactions happened simultaneously. My thoughts and memories about bombings created a very lifelike illusion that triggered a response in my body as I dived for cover.

Yes, when I was threatened, that flash of adrenaline-pumping fear and quick reactions were, of course, necessary to survive. However, some 40 years later, when the sound was a car backfiring, such physical responses no longer served me. Since then, I have noted that my reaction reduces greatly in a calm state of mind.

So it's important to note that you do not need to be afraid of your experience or your thoughts as you have the power to choose whether to give a thought life or not. I'm sure you have had a crazy thought once or twice in your life!

I remember psychiatrist Dr Bill Pettit sharing an experience he had one day driving home from work. He stopped at traffic lights, and as people were crossing the road in front of his car, he had a random thought: "If I accelerated right now, I could take out at least 10 people!" Thankfully, he knew it was a crazy thought, which he obviously did not act on. Instead, he knew to look inside for wisdom in the moment and realised he was exhausted and needed to slow down.

Feelings can take the form of emotions or sensations. Thoughts and feelings occur simultaneously and cannot be separated; doing so would be like trying to separate the mind from the body; they go hand in hand.

Emotions such as fear, anger, anxiety, depression or misery, or on the other hand, joy, peace and love, can each be felt in our bodies. We are often so caught up in our heads, consumed by our thoughts and thinking, that we are unaware of what is happening beneath our skin. We tend to categorise our emotions as good or bad. But what if all of them are love 'disguised' because, whether they feel good or not, they are all guiding us into balance, towards health? The same can be said for each sensation we feel in the body, including uncomfortable sensations such as tightness, tension, bracing, or even pain.

If I think back to before the episode of acute back pain that I had, my body had been speaking to me long before my back went. In the months prior, I had not only lost my two beautiful Labrador dogs – both 15 years old, who succumbed to old age – but I had also lost my father-in-law, who passed away only 10 weeks after a terminal diagnosis. All this grief was held in my body, and its whispers were clearly not getting my attention, so my body had to scream at me instead.

I had foolishly chosen to ignore my body, remaining instead in my head with my thoughts and thinking (personal mind).

This pattern continued even when I was in extreme pain; I stayed in my head, trying to fix my body, ignoring the wisdom that lay inside, obscured by the noise of my own thinking.

> *"If the only thing people learned was not to be afraid of their experience, that alone would change the world."*
>
> Michael Neill

When we understand how our experience is created from moment to moment, we see that we don't have to be afraid of feelings of sadness, regret, or anger; we begin to see them for what they are – simply thoughts in the moment.

Every feeling has a thought at its core, and when we give a particular thought some attention, it acts like a magnet, attracting other thoughts and building momentum and strength. If we recognise each thought for what it is – just a thought – and choose not to add weight to it, it will pass, and so will the associated feelings.

> *"Every single thought that we have that we give life to either promotes health or it promotes dis-ease."*
>
> Dr Bill Pettit

Until recently, I innocently believed that all of my thoughts were true. It's only now that I realise I have a choice to act on a thought, to believe it or let it pass. Thought is a creative gift we can use in any way we choose. Remember, a thought only has as much power as you choose to give it.

When a random thought pops into our mind, when we don't grab hold of it, it will pass by, just like the clouds in the sky; they are always on the move. But we humans tend to grab thoughts, creating a thought thunderstorm that consumes us. We become so convinced that the storm is real when, in reality, it's only ever a very clever illusion.

My Story

Have you ever been getting ready to go out somewhere when you look in the mirror and think, "Oh my goodness, I've put on some weight recently!" This happened to me last summer when I was on holiday with my two grown-up kids and my husband, Peter. Just before we went out for an evening meal, I glanced in the mirror, felt that my dress was a bit tight and thought, "Oh dear!" and my mood sank.

We dined in a beautiful restaurant perched on top of a cliff, overlooking the sea with its deep blue and green hues and the gentle sound of the waves caressing the pebbles below. Despite the stunning location and having precious time with our kids before they both headed for Australia later that year, I spent the whole evening feeling uncomfortable in my own skin. That one thought had developed into a storm of negative thoughts about my body. In a low mood, I listened to my thoughts, and boy, did those thoughts look real. My self-critical thoughts were stickier than superglue, and I was convinced they were true. If my thoughts ever created how I experienced my body, it was certainly in that moment.

"Thought creates our world and then says, 'I didn't do it!'"

David Bohm (1917-1992)
American theoretical physicist

I knew my thinking was creating self-loathing, but knowing this didn't make it any less sticky in that moment. I could hear my mentor, Mavis Karn, say, "Know not to trust your thinking when you are in a low mood." But it looked real! That's what the power of Thought does – it looks real, particularly so when you are in a low mood.

Fast-forward a few days, my mood lifted, and I was able to see the mirage. I happened to be reading Thomas M. Kelly's 'Upside-Down and Backwards' and it hit me: I have spent years trying different diets and buying ridiculous amounts of nice clothes to try to control my insecure thinking. All along, I hadn't understood that thinking was the source of my emotional pain; I had spent energy and expense reaching outside of myself for solutions. This had been my coping strategy in attempting to minimise my pain. I had been searching 'out there' for a source of relief, but it was futile.

I innocently lived in the illusion that I needed another beautiful piece of clothing to feel good and comfortable in my body. This need for something new led me to misguidedly think self-image and confidence were tied to 'stuff out there.'

My insecurity and need to wear something that might make me feel good were products of my own personal thinking. My urge to buy another lovely item was another seductive personal thought that came to mind, particularly when I felt low about myself. All my shopping was an attempt to quiet my compelling, sticky and habitual thoughts about being insecure and hating myself.

It's time to see where those feelings were coming from. Whatever I am feeling is always and only determined by how I use the power of Mind, Consciousness, and Thought. Knowing this in my heart and not just in my head means I am no longer a victim; I can let go of feeling insecure. Indeed, my security and confidence have been hiding in plain sight all this time; it's only now, as my personal mind clears and the mist lifts, that I trust I can find true and lasting peace of mind.

> "Thoughts have no power of their own,
> only that which you give them."
>
> Sydney Banks

I have paid too much attention to how I look in the mirror, thinking it defines me rather than listening to my body and trusting the wisdom within. I have all the confidence I need; it's just got covered up by the layers of thinking, judgement and beliefs I have developed over time.

Common sense tells me to actually wear the beautiful clothes already in my wardrobe – all the items I've never had the confidence to wear until now – because they are beautiful, not because they will make me any more gorgeous. I have a choice about how I experience my body in this moment. So, I choose not to ruminate, contaminate, or judge; instead, I trust my guide inside to nudge me towards curiosity, compassion, and love for myself.

Today, I walked into a restaurant to meet family and friends, wearing my vintage handcrafted Indian wrap skirt in stunning shades of turquoise, green, and red, which I had never worn before. I wore my vivid gold and turquoise drop earrings, hidden away in my jewellery box, because they might draw attention to me. It felt good to allow that bohemian part of myself outside in the daylight. I walked taller with my shoulders back, despite thoughts that I wasn't enough crossing the screen of my mind; I recognised them as old judgements; I blessed them and sent them on their way. I walked in beauty.

What does my story about body image and clothing have to do with chronic pain?

I am making the point that when we struggle with chronic pain, it's good to remember that in a low mood, it's easy to slip into a cycle of worry. Anxious and fearful thoughts then add fuel to the fire of chronic pain. In other words, chronic emotional pain exacerbates chronic physical pain.

We each have hidden habits of thought that we innocently pick up, but these habitual patterns do not have to dominate us. Our habitual thoughts shout the loudest and tend to rule us, especially when we are in a low mood. Often, the quieter, softer voice inside our head speaks with wisdom. The louder voice obscures our wisdom, but we usually see more clearly when we have a clear mind and can let go of the noise.

I am sure you have experienced this, for example, when you lose your keys and desperately retrace your steps to find where you hid them! Giving up, you put the kettle on, and as you stand waiting for it to boil, your mind quiets down. Suddenly, a new thought pops up, and you can remember now exactly where you left them.

Now, when my back feels tight and stiff, instead of listening to my loud habitual thoughts such as "Oh no, my back is going to go out again," I listen for the whispers of wisdom: "You are trying to squeeze too many patients into your diary at the moment. Slow down."

Once we see that our feelings are love in disguise, we hear our body's wisdom, which tells us when we are off base or that our thinking is not to be trusted. We each have a built-in GPS that guides us back to balance – if only we would listen. When we lose a light-hearted feeling or restful well-being, it's a sign to slow down!

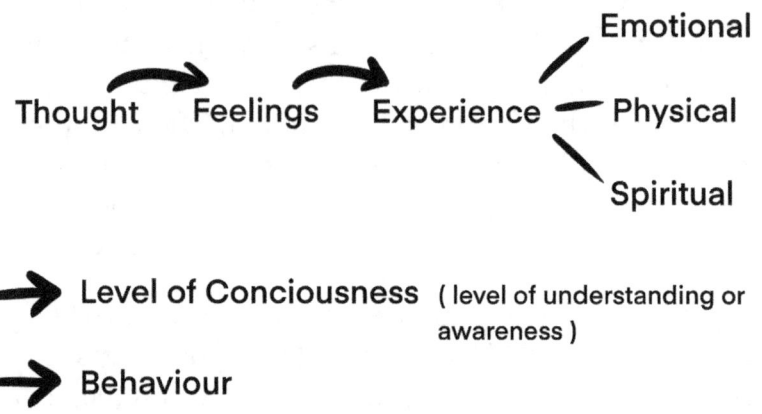

→ **Level of Conciousness** (level of understanding or awareness)

→ **Behaviour**

When you have an anxious thought, you feel anxiety somewhere in your body. You may feel it in the pit of your stomach, or in your shoulders or neck. When you have an angry thought, perhaps you feel it in the clench of your jaw or a tightness in your chest. If you react from this place of feeling, your behaviour will be fuelled with anger, perhaps causing you to do something you later regret.

We are designed to feel all feelings, yet we spend time and energy fighting the ones we don't like – those that make us feel afraid. But our feelings are not the enemy. They are simply energy taking form in the mind and body, passing through like waves. When we understand that they are made of thought, we no longer need to fix or change them. Feelings are not the problem; they are part of the human experience.

Yet, when I was in the depths of my back pain, I didn't see it that way. I knew, intellectually, that the body is designed to heal within six to eight weeks after an injury. And yet, as the months passed and my pain remained, I was fearful. My mind was spinning with anxious thoughts such as "Why isn't this going away? What if it never does?" and I couldn't see a way out.

Looking back now, I realise I was caught in a snowstorm of my own making, like a shaken snow globe where everything is swirling, chaotic, and unclear. When our minds are full of fearful thinking, we can't see the truth: all pain is real, but suffering comes from the meaning we attach to it.

The body always tells the truth. You can't sneak a thought past it.

But the good news? Just as the snow in a shaken globe eventually settles, so too does the mind – if we stop stirring it up. And when the mind settles, the body can finally follow.

If emotions are energy that takes form in the mind and the body, could my thoughts and emotions be taking form as pain?

Key Takeaways

◊ **Personal Story of Pain and Recovery:** My intense episode of back pain following emotional stress and grief, highlighting the interplay between physical symptoms and psychological factors.

◊ **The Mind-Body Connection:** Thoughts directly impact bodily sensations. Chronic pain often stems from psychological patterns rather than structural causes.

◊ **Thoughts Shape Our Reality:** The power of Thought determines emotions and perceptions so recognising them as transient can restore clarity and peace.

◊ **Listening to Inner Wisdom:** The body offers signals to guide balance/well-being. Connecting to the quiet mind and trusting inner wisdom, leads us to deeper healing and resilience.

Chapter 6

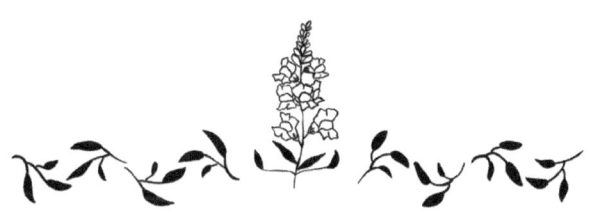

The Feeling is Foolproof

*"Our feelings are a barometer of how our **thoughts** are being utilised."*

Sydney Banks

HUMANS SPEND MOST OF their time in their heads, ignoring their bodies. I know I did, until Myofascial Release Therapy opened my eyes to how I was bracing and holding tension in my body. I learned to drop out of my head and into my body, feeling my way into healing. The more I listened, the more I saw that feelings, sensations and emotions were not burdens to suppress but whispers of wisdom from the universe, leading me towards healing.

The Cost of Ignoring Our Feelings

We are taught from an early age to suppress emotions and override sensations, particularly those deemed negative or inconvenient. We learn to silence our inner experience, stuffing emotions down in an attempt to maintain composure and meet expectations. Over time, this detachment from our feelings severs the connection between mind, body and spirit, creating a disconnection from the truth within us.

We grow up believing it's unsafe to feel everything we are feeling. The fast pace of life leaves little space for real-time feelings, so instead, they are labelled as an inconvenience. We pretend that "All is well" and "I'm fine." Meanwhile, we choose to numb or bury our feelings deep into the cells of our bodies. We hide things from others and ourselves because we think it's easier to ignore or suppress our feelings rather than to face them. But could it be that feelings are part of our design, and here for a reason: to serve as a portal to our body's wisdom?

My Story

> In 2000, while in the foothills of the Himalayas, I contracted viral meningitis. What followed was a 15-year struggle with chronic pain, fatigue and various diagnoses from post-viral fatigue to chronic fatigue and eventually to fibromyalgia. I was balancing a demanding career and raising young children, telling myself I had no time to slow down. I ignored my body's pleas for attention, pushing forward with sheer determination. I didn't have

time to listen to my body or deal with the emotions of being completely overwhelmed. I often came home after a busy day at work feeling worn ragged, with raw emotions – fear and frustration bubbling beneath the surface. I was exhausted after work and had little energy left for my family. I told myself I had to succeed in my career at all costs.

It never occurred to me that the feelings I was repressing were trying to express themselves through my pain. Looking back, I see that I innocently and stubbornly ignored the love letters from my body.

I grew up believing that you should just get on with it. If you felt emotions rising, you shoved them back down and pushed on through whatever situation you found yourself in. Perhaps this belief was a remnant of growing up during The Troubles in Northern Ireland. It was a time when fear was ever present, yet rarely acknowledged.

Reconnecting to the Body's Wisdom

In 2015, I discovered Myofascial Release, a therapy that led me back into my body. I began to listen – truly listen – to the sensations and emotions that arose, recognising them as messages rather than problems to fix. (See my first book, *Finding Mystery Within*.)

I have come to understand that our body's signals are not random. They are precise, intelligent messages designed to bring us back into alignment. When we ignore them, they intensify, much like a child tugging at a parent's sleeve for attention. If we continue to dismiss them, they escalate into physical discomfort, chronic pain, or illness.

What if it's safe to feel and it's safe to cry? All too often, we deny or control our felt experience, but what if this behaviour smothers the voice of our soul, severing the link between us and our body? There is a Divinity, a wisdom within that speaks to us, but we silence it. The static of our judging thoughts obscures the gentle, wise whisper of wisdom.

By not listening to or avoiding our feelings, sensations, and emotions, we betray our bodies and abandon the Truth that lives in each of us.

As I grasped the importance of trusting the feelings and sensations that arose, I learned to feel and breathe again, fully entering life. I spent too long holding my breath, becoming invisible and not feeling since I was a little girl. It was exhausting to suppress and hold down all my feelings. Now, when I see that my breathing becomes shallow or when I catch myself holding my breath or clenching my jaw, I know I need to listen to the signal from my body that I'm off-centre. I have lost sight of the ever-present wisdom. When I take a deep breath, feel and get curious, I can see which thoughts I'm paying too much attention to.

Living an embodied life invites us to trust the wisdom that arises, wisdom felt through the body. So, instead of resisting what arises, we trust that we have a place of peace within where optimal healing can be found. Rather than trying to get rid of dis-ease, we can find a place of ease with dis-ease. A place of trust that healing will come.

Life seeks to heal itself when we go with the flow, saying yes to everything that shows up. As we orientate towards wholeness, we see something new needs to be embraced and included.

The Power of Awareness

My Story

A few months ago, I was invited to be a guest on Paola Royal's podcast, Your Life... but easier. My initial reaction was resistance – a mix of fear and self-doubt. As the interview date approached, my body responded; I became aware that I was clenching my teeth at night, waking each morning with sensitive teeth and pinched skin inside my cheeks. The day before, my stomach felt nauseous, and my lower back began to tighten and ache. I might have ignored or dismissed these symptoms in the past, but instead, I paused and listened. I sat with these feelings, resisting the temptation to ignore or shove them down. I allowed them space. I acknowledged my nervousness without judgement. Instead of fearing the fear, I observed it. As a result, my body softened, and I met the experience with calm curiosity rather than resistance. The interview came and went, and I showed up fully present rather than consumed by my thoughts.

Trusting the Intelligence Behind Life

Our feelings are not here to harm us but to guide us. Instead of resisting pain or discomfort, we can trust them as a doorway to deeper healing. When we shift from fighting our experience to embracing it, we work with life rather than against it.

So much of our suffering comes from the belief that life is happening to us rather than through us. We attribute our emotions to external circumstances, believing that other people, situations, or past events are responsible for how we feel. But in truth, our feelings arise from within, shaped by our thoughts in the moment. When we understand this, we no longer feel like victims of life. But we begin to trust the feelings that arise and see that we are constantly being guided back home – to the truth within us.

Healing is not about eliminating symptoms but about understanding them. So, instead of resisting discomfort, we meet it with openness, and rather than fearing illness, we see it as an invitation to deepen our relationship with ourselves. When we embrace our feelings and sensations as part of our innate intelligence, we step into a deeper trust – trust that life is unfolding exactly as it should, trust that we are always being guided, and trust that healing is not about fixing ourselves but about remembering who we truly are.

Feelings are not obstacles; they are signposts. They are not something to be feared; they are a call to presence. They are not random; they are the universe whispering to us, inviting us to listen.

So, to sum up: When we embrace our feelings and live from a place of love, we widen and deepen our embodiment. We return to love; we come home. We understand that feelings are trying to keep us safe. They are not something to be fixed. They are messengers guiding us back home, an invitation to open something new and fresh rather than to contract in judgement.

If thoughts are the language of the mind and feelings are the language of the body, then how we think and feel creates our state of being.

Key Takeaways

◊ **Feelings as Guides, Not Burdens:** Our emotions, sensations, and bodily signals are messages of wisdom guiding us towards healing; listening to them fosters alignment.

◊ **The Cost of Ignoring Our Feelings:** Unprocessed feelings don't disappear; they manifest as physical tension, pain, or illness.

◊ **Reconnecting to the Body's Wisdom:** By shifting to awareness, bodily sensations are seen as invitations to heal rather than problems to fix.

◊ **Trusting the Intelligence of Life:** Life is not happening to us but through us. When we trust our feelings, we embrace discomfort as a path to deeper self-understanding and healing.

Chapter 7

This is the Age of Well-Being

THE AGE OF WELL-BEING marks a profound cultural shift in which holistic physical, mental, emotional, and spiritual health takes centre stage. We are moving away from reactive, symptom-focused healthcare towards a proactive approach that nurtures healing from the inside out. This evolution is underpinned by breakthroughs in neuroscience and psychology and insights drawn from ancient wisdom traditions, all of which recognise the profound connection between mind, body, and spirit.

Over the years, I have witnessed this shift first-hand – not only through my work with chronic pain patients but also in the world at large. Today, science is beginning to acknowledge that our experience of life is not merely physical but also deeply spiritual. My book reflects this emerging understanding, as I view chronic pain and suffering as phenomena shaped by Mind, Consciousness, and Thought. We are collectively evolving beyond the limitations of the biomedical model, gradually embracing how our state of mind, emotions, and sense of purpose play essential roles in healing.

Science and spirituality are not at odds; they complement one another in explaining the nature of reality, consciousness, and healing. Many scientists are speaking of this necessary shift in awareness. As quantum physicist and author of *The Self-Aware Universe*, Amit Goswami reminds us, "*Consciousness is the ground of all being. Science must evolve to include it, not ignore it.*"

Similarly, Gregg Braden, geologist and author of *The Divine Matrix*, observes that, "*The bridge between science and spirituality is consciousness. When we become aware of our thoughts, emotions, and intentions, we can change our reality.*"

Even Sydney Banks has noted that the power of Thought is the bridge between the formless Mind and the form – the Body. This raises an essential question for each of us: What does this shift mean for my personal healing journey and how can I actively engage with it?

Becoming Conscious of the Role of Thought

If this book offers one insight that has the potential to transform your life, it is the realisation of the profound influence your thoughts have on your health and well-being. Your habitual thought patterns – often rooted in past experiences, limiting beliefs, or unexamined narratives of pain – shape the reality you live each day.

In the previous chapter, I recognised fear as a dominant, deeply ingrained pattern that can cause me to suffer. Indeed, thoughts can move so quickly that we often don't notice them before the emotion hits. This is especially true in PTSD (chronic activation of the stress response via thoughts about past events stored in our memories), where an innocent trigger can make the past feel vividly present. Yet, the past no longer exists – only our thinking creates such a lifelike mirage that our body has no choice but to respond.

Dr Bill Pettit shares a powerful example. A former soldier attending a conference in Barcelona unknowingly arrived on a national holiday, where fireworks exploded in celebration. The sudden noise triggered an immediate physiological reaction – his heart raced, he broke into a cold sweat, and his legs gave way. Yet, because of his grounding in the Three Principles, he recognised that this was a mirage created by Thought. The fear felt real, but he knew he didn't have to be afraid of his experience. By finding a quiet mind, his body naturally followed, and the symptoms passed.

Many of us unknowingly disrupt our body's natural chemistry with habitual thought patterns – whether these are rooted in fear, anxiety, worry, depression or persistent pain. The key to healing isn't found in analysing these thoughts, but in allowing the mind to quieten enough to allow natural healing to occur. No matter what your habitual thought pattern is, the answer to breaking it is spiritual!

The Bridge Between Science and Spirituality

In her beautiful book *The Awakened Brain*, Dr Lisa Miller reveals how spirituality protects against mental suffering. Believe it or not, a spiritual brain can be seen on MRI findings! Miller's research shows that when someone places low importance on spirituality, their scan shows a few intermittent tiny red patches, which are associated with health. However, for those who place high importance on spirituality, their brain scans have vast swaths of red. These findings suggest that the brains of more spiritually-orientated people are healthier and more robust.

Spirituality isn't only about religion – it's about recognising our connection to something greater than ourselves. Spiritual consciousness can be seen as something beyond spirituality. It begins when we realise we are creating everything with Thought. When we know we are creating our experience with Thought, we see we have the power to choose our response to every circumstance and relationship.

When we know we are creative energy in motion, a conscious super-intelligence, and choosing how we are experiencing life, we can then use our awakened brain to live in an optimally healthy way, no matter what physical limitations we may be dealing with. Even someone with severe physical limitations – for example, someone who lives with quadriplegia – has the capacity to experience joy, love and creativity or pain, suffering and despair… and everything in between due to spiritual consciousness [an awakened brain]. Spiritual consciousness shows us that the power to choose rests on how we use the power of Divine Thought – which thoughts we choose to bring to life.

Dr Miller continues, *"Each of us has an awakened brain. Each of us is endowed with a natural capacity to perceive a greater reality and consciously connect to the life force that moves in, through and around us."* She states that our brains are wired to perceive that which uplifts, illuminates, and heals! Spiritual experience is a vital yet overlooked component of healing. But it's a choice to enter into a dialogue with the loving, guiding universe.

Our Feeling State Has the Greatest Impact on Healing

As a newly graduated physiotherapist in 1990, I never would have imagined that researchers would one day investigate the effects our thoughts and feelings have on our healing, health, and well-being. The implications of this shift are far-reaching. Imagine a state of being where our feelings of joy, gratitude and acceptance enrich our inner lives and have measurable, positive impacts on our physical health.

As research in this field rapidly grows, the results point to how feelings of joy, bliss, gratitude, or acceptance influence us at a physiological level. This suggests that this set of feelings reduce stress, improve heart health, boost immune function, release endorphins, increase longevity, enhance brain function, and even relieve pain.

Could it be that joy and bliss don't only feel good but that they have a measurable, positive impact on our physical health and even aid healing? If so, then it also makes sense that, on the flip side, not only does our brain chemistry change if we become consumed with anxious or depressed thinking, but so too does our body's physiology change over time with the kind of thinking we are living in. Depression is often labelled as a 'chemical imbalance' in the brain, but what if that chemical imbalance was created by us innocently believing our negative or depressing thoughts?

If our life experience arises from the energy of our thoughts being translated into a physical experience through consciousness, then depression, anxiety, and persistent pain do not exist without Thought and the way we think. Understanding that thinking will change, offers us hope that we don't have to permanently stay stuck in a cycle of habitual, repetitive, negative thinking. Just as thinking changes throughout the day, so will our thinking change from moment to moment if we allow it.

My Story

A few years ago, I was caught in a cycle of thinking that kept me stuck in a place of pain and resentment because of someone else's actions, or so I believed. Then, a new thought arose during a quiet walk with my dogs. "I am only a victim for as long as I keep choosing to believe those victim thoughts!"

Where did that new thought come from? It wasn't something I consciously generated. It was wisdom breaking through the noise. It was as if someone had shaken me out of the victimhood movie that kept playing on repeat in my head, and I suddenly could see where my suffering was coming from — from my thoughts about the situation. I saw that I could substitute any belief into that sentence.

I am only 'insecure' for as long as I keep choosing to believe insecure thoughts about myself.

I am only 'broken' for as long as I keep choosing to believe thoughts about being broken.

I am only ……. for as long as I keep choosing to believe thoughts about being ……….

We all innocently get caught up in a story created by our thoughts. When a thought enters our conscious awareness, it feels like reality, so we tend to believe it.

In his groundbreaking book, *Quantum Healing: Exploring the Frontiers of Mind/Body Medicine*, Deepak Chopra says, *"Every cell in your body is eavesdropping on your thoughts."*

Bill Pettit clarifies that this only applies to the thoughts we pay attention to and give life to with our consciousness. Sydney Banks observed that thoughts that pass through the body-mind without being juiced by personal consciousness are harmless.

Anxiety exists because we pay attention to anxious thoughts. Pain persists because we focus on painful thoughts. What we nurture in our mind grows. But when we see how our experience is created – once we are spiritually conscious – we open the door to something new. We all know how loud habitual thinking can be, obscuring our wisdom or common sense. Wisdom is primarily quiet, soft, and gentle, and can only be heard with a clear mind. All too often, it gets buried under the noise of our personal thinking. The soul's wisdom emerges when the mind quiets, guiding us towards healing. Sometimes, when we don't listen, our soul finds louder ways to get our attention – through symptoms, emotions, or persistent thoughts.

> *"When the mind quiets, love reveals itself as the constant beneath the noise of thought."*
>
> Mark Howard, PhD

Once we truly grasp the power of our thoughts on our bodies, we step into a whole new paradigm of healing – one in which we are no longer prisoners of our thinking but creators of our experience. In this realisation, we find freedom.

Key Takeaways

◊ **Holistic Health Shift:** The cultural transition from reactive, purely biomedical care to a proactive, holistic approach, integrating physical, mental, emotional and spiritual well-being.

◊ **Power of Thought:** Our habitual thought patterns shape our experiences of pain and suffering; awareness and change in thought can lead to healing.

◊ **Science Meets Spirituality:** Science is beginning to acknowledge and incorporate the role of consciousness and spirituality, bridging the gap between scientific and the spiritual.

◊ **Emotional Impact on Healing:** Positive emotions lift our mental state and have tangible, beneficial effects on our physical health.

Chapter 8

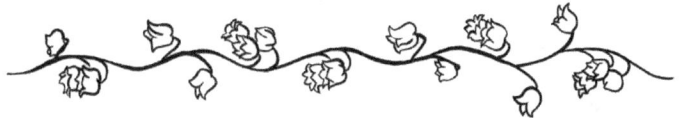

Understanding Pain

NOW THAT WE HAVE SEEN how our moment-to-moment experience is created, let's talk about pain. In the first couple of chapters, I referred to the fact that for centuries, we held the belief that pain is simply a result of stimulation of the sensory receptors in the body. However, this purely biomedical model has gradually been found lacking. We now realise that psychological, cognitive, emotional, and spiritual factors are at play. Pain is not simply a signal that something is wrong in the body, but rather a protective response generated by our mind's response to perceived threats. In other words, thoughts and thinking contribute to the experience of pain.

For those of you who are now saying, "You haven't seen how bad my scan is!", I need to point out that pain is an unreliable indicator of what is happening in our bodies. In a podcast interview with Dr Rangan Chatterjee (Episode 310, *Feel Better, Live More* podcast), Dr Howard Schubiner shares some incredible statistics:

- There is no physical cause for chronic neck and back pain in 88% of people who report it

- MRI scans show that of:
    - 30-year-olds with NO pain – 30% have bulging disc and 40% have degenerative disc disease
    - 50-year-olds with NO pain – 60% have bulging discs, 30% have herniated discs and 80% have degenerative disc disease
    - 60-year-olds with NO pain – 90% have abnormalities present

So…

A disc bulge does not equal pain!

Disc degeneration does not equal pain!

These are normal findings on a scan.

Scan results can fill you with fear and avoidance, which only serve to keep you stuck in a cycle of chronic pain. Suppose you freak out and panic over your scan results. In that case, you will have a powerful emotional response, causing you to overprotect your body, and the nervous system response will create a massive sensitisation.

Trust me when I say the body is incredible and way beyond our understanding. Pain is not as simple as cause and effect. There is no single cause of pain; it is a complex combination of factors – physical, biological, emotional, psychological, and spiritual – after all, we are physical, emotional, and spiritual beings.

Despite severe injury, there are vast recorded examples when pain is not switched on. Imagine spraining your ankle badly while trying to cross a busy road while a huge lorry hurtles towards you. You would keep moving while your brain shuts off pain in an attempt to save your life!

Pain is a multifaceted experience. Our beliefs can influence it; that is, the story someone else has told us or something we believe to be true. For example, a doctor tells you that you have the neck of an 80-year-old, or you have a "slipped disc" (there is no such thing as a slipped disc by the way!). What does that language do for you? It often leads you to a place where your thoughts spiral out of control. Also, believe it or not, someone with low self-worth can influence their experience of persistent pain.

Smudging

Have you ever heard the word *homunculus*? It's a Latin word that means 'little man', and it is used in neuroanatomy to denote the sensory map of the human body on the cerebral cortex/brain. (See the image below.) So when a person is experiencing a sore knee, for example, that part of the homunculus lights up on the corresponding part of the brain.

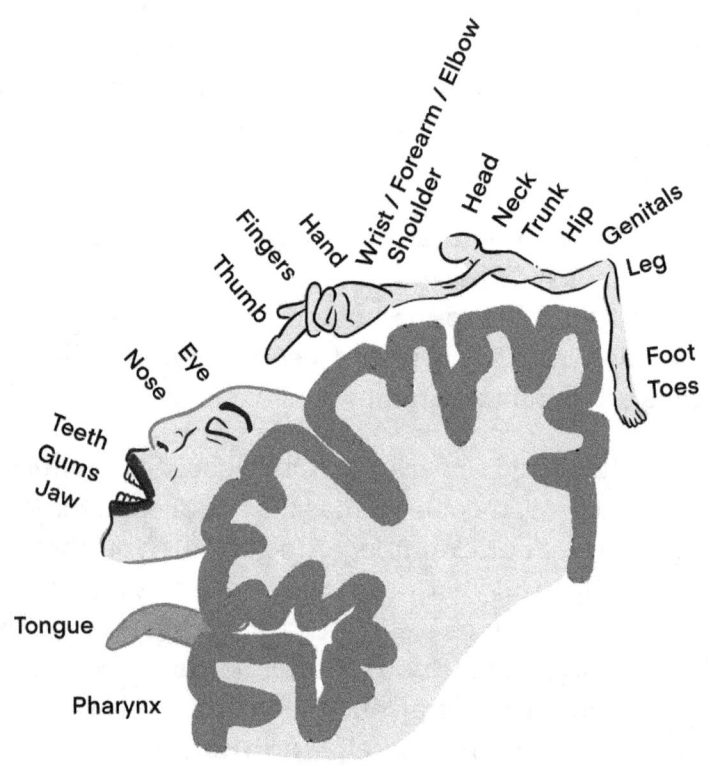

Smudging is a description of the changes in the brain that occur when someone experiences chronic pain. For example, when a person experiences pain in a specific body part, such as the knee, adjacent body parts in the homunculus may also offer the perception of pain. I like to think of it as ink spreading on a piece of blotting paper. This means that the size of the area in the cerebral cortex that usually represents the knee grows and becomes more extensive. We can innocently cause this by rubbing our knee every time we think about how sore it is or even in anticipation of it being painful. Constantly massaging and stimulating all the sensory nerve endings in the knee increases its sensitivity, and representation on the homunculus map of our cortex gets bigger.

Smudging and crosstalk are common concepts in chronic pain and can even occur without tissue injury; in other words, once the injury has healed, the neural pathways in the brain remain on high alert. Research shows that the neurocircuitry for an injury can continue long after the injury has healed, and what causes it to continue is the memory of the injury, the fear of it. Other stressors then tend to switch it on, as the neurocircuitry becomes a default pathway, easily triggered by stress or anxiety. This default pathway gets reinforced over time by our fearful thinking.

So the lens of judgements we look through, or beliefs we hold dear, can cause smudging of the neural circuitry, keeping memories alive. The memory of the pain traps us in a fear loop, which perpetuates our pain. If you've ever experienced severe acute pain following an injury, it takes very little to throw you back into that memory of the past.

There are often deep emotional connections where a specific memory can trigger old pain. In other words, a significant emotional upset, such as the death of a loved one, can trigger an old pain pattern. This is very common in low back pain patients. Indeed, neuroscience shows that emotions and stress activate the same part of the brain as physical injuries. Therefore, emotional pain can manifest as physical pain.

Dr Lorimer Moseley provides a brilliant example in his TEDx Adelaide Talk, 'Why Things Hurt.' Please listen to it as he is an incredibly gifted communicator, but I'll share it here in my own words for now.

[www.youtube.com/watch?v=gwd-wLdIHjs]

Eight years ago, Lorimer was walking in the bush in Australia wearing a sarong when he felt something touch the outside of his left leg. His brain interpreted this as not dangerous because, as a boy, he had spent many years walking through the bush, having his legs scratched by twigs and causing no harm. But on this particular occasion, he had just been bitten by an Eastern brown snake, which is highly poisonous. This was the last thing he remembered. He was fortunate to survive.

Six months later, he was walking in the bush again when he felt something touch the outside of his left leg, and immediately he felt white hot searing pain shooting up his leg. This time, his brain interpreted it as DANGER! The brain registered he was in the same situation as when he had last felt this sensation on the outside of his left leg. His severe pain continued until his friend pointed out he had just scraped the outside of his leg on a twig. His brain knew that when he'd had a similar experience, he had almost died.

This anecdote demonstrates that pain is an illusion 100% of the time, created not by your body's tissues but by your brain to protect you.

Understanding how the mind works is crucial, and I'm not talking about the brain here. That's why I've spent the last few chapters diving into this subject. The brain is the chemical, anatomical structure inside our skull, whereas the mind is spiritual. As Sydney Banks says in *The Enlightened Gardener*, *"The brain, by itself, lacks the power to think; just as a refrigerator must have electricity to function, so the brain must have Mind as a power source to make it work."*

I often see patients experiencing pain long after an initial injury has healed. Their chronic pain comes from the thinking they hold about the initial injury and from innocently maintaining pain habits, such as reduced activity levels, movement avoidance and bracing. And hear me when I say, "No judgement here!" It happened to me too!

My Story

When I injured my back, as described in Chapter 5, I suffered excruciating, crippling pain and got stuck on the kitchen floor, unable to move or breathe. I held and moved my body in ways that I thought would protect me from experiencing that pain again. The only problem was that I got stuck in that bracing pattern, which led the neural pathways in my brain to become overreactive and hypersensitive when I moved in certain ways. The slightest twinge elicited feelings and memories of the original injury.

About two months after my initial episode had fully resolved, here's what happened:

I was in the bathroom and turned to my right, bending over slightly to flush the toilet and bang; I felt a sharp stabbing pain followed by my back going into a complete spasm. I felt a stab of fear. I thought, "I can't do this again, not another four months of this pain!"

I caught myself and thought, "No, I'm not going down that rabbit hole of fearful thinking again. **I am sore but safe.** *I am going to be OK."*

The pain lasted 48 hours and went as quickly as it had come.

A sensitised nervous system can flag up a historically sensitised area to get us to slow down or stop. An old pain can arise when fighting an infection, such as a cold or flu. I saw this a lot during COVID or post-vaccine – old symptoms would flare up, such as sciatica or concussion.

Imagine a well-worn rut in a muddy path that you are cycling along. Your bicycle wheel always finds a rut, so staying on that particular trajectory is more straightforward than finding a new, less worn pathway. This is what happens in our brains when we experience chronic pain; those well-worn pain pathways become our default pathway whenever our brain interprets any situation as DANGEROUS. The pain pathways in the brain become so easily triggered that any threat, such as an anxious thought, worry, or stress, can trigger a familiar, well-worn path, causing us to experience more pain.

This demonstrates that our psychology influences our experience of pain, i.e. patients with stress, anxiety, depression, adverse childhood events (ACEs), or trauma have less ability to inhibit their pain. Their anxious, fearful thoughts about their pain cause neuroplastic changes in the brain tissues.

> Neuroplastic is the medical term for oversensitive pain pathways. This means they tend to have a decreased threshold because they are stuck in 'fight or flight,' so their body perceives threats 24/7.

The Fight-or-Flight Response

The fight-or-flight response is a natural survival mechanism that has saved countless lives. Here's how it affects the body:

- **Increased adrenaline/epinephrine:** Raises heart rate, boosts blood flow to large muscles for escape, and heightens alertness.

- **Increased cortiso:** Speeds up metabolism for quick energy.

- **Increased glucose:** Provides immediate fuel.

- **Inhibited insulin secretion:** Keeps glucose readily available.

- **Slowed digestion:** Redirects energy to essential functions.

- **Rapid, shallow breathing:** Enhances oxygen intake.

- **Weakened immune response and slower healing:** Energy is conserved for survival.

- **Hypercoagulable blood:** Reduces excessive bleeding from injuries.

These responses are beneficial in the short term. However, the body is only designed to sustain them for up to 30 minutes per day. When stress becomes chronic, the prolonged activation of this system disrupts the body's ability to return to a natural, balanced state. This can lead to inflammation, digestive issues, skin conditions, reproductive problems, diabetes, heart disease, strokes, and blood clots.

Stress isn't just triggered by physical threats – it can also be activated by worry, overthinking, guilt, resentment, anger, grief, and chronic negative thought patterns.

Chronic pain causes 'central sensitisation' or 'neuroplastic pain' which explains why some people have a disproportionate pain response through no fault of their own.

Interestingly, Dr Bill Pettit has observed that self-forgiveness and forgiving others play a crucial role in resolving pain.

All pain is real. It is the brain's response to something threatening or dangerous; it's a danger alarm system, not just a tissue injury alarm system. Pain is experienced when our brain perceives credible evidence of danger, inferring the need to protect.

There is a well-documented case of a builder who fell from some scaffolding, landing feet first onto a six-inch nail, piercing through his boot. He took one look at the protruding nail and cried out in pain. An ambulance was called, and he was given gas and air (nitrous oxide) for pain relief on his way to the hospital. Once he was safely in the Emergency Room, doctors and nurses carefully removed his boot, only to discover the nail went cleanly through the space between his toes, causing no actual injury, not even piercing his skin!

Sometimes, this protective system can become turned up and edgy.

But the good news is that when you understand why you hurt, you may hurt less.

Key Takeaways

◊ **Pain as a Multifaceted Experience:** Pain is a complex interplay of physical, emotional, psychological, and spiritual factors.

◊ **The Role of Perception in Pain:** Fear and negative beliefs about 'normal' findings can lead to chronic pain through heightened sensitivity and overprotection by the nervous system.

◊ **Neuroplasticity and Pain Sensitisation:** Smudging, where neural pathways become hypersensitive due to fear, memory, or stress, creates a cycle where emotional triggers or past injuries perpetuate pain.

◊ **Breaking the Pain Cycle:** Understanding the psychological and neuroplastic nature of pain empowers individuals to disrupt well-worn pain pathways and foster recovery.

Chapter 9

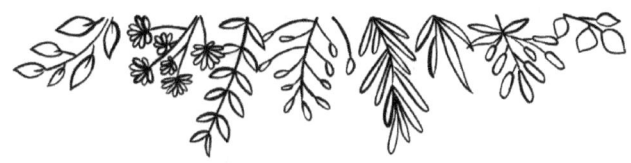

Re-Thinking Pain

AS WE REACH THE HALFWAY point of this book, I invite you to pause and reflect. Before we move forward, let's revisit four key insights we've already explored. These insights are essential in deepening our understanding of persistent pain and reshaping our experience of it. Below is a recap of what we have covered so far.

- Pain protects us and promotes healing.
- Persisting pain overprotects us and prevents recovery.
- Many factors influence pain.
- Understanding the inside-out nature of life.

Pain Protects Us and Promotes Healing

Every occurrence of pain (acute or chronic) protects us from what the brain 'perceives' as danger. A sprained ankle creates pain, which causes us to avoid moving through our full range of motion because it hurts. This temporary immobilisation allows the damaged ligaments to heal, which is how pain promotes healing.

When we are injured, our pain settings ramp up straight away; pain prevents the mechanical forces from exceeding the injured tissue's strength in its current state, thereby preventing further injury and allowing healing. Our body has an innate capacity to heal itself – it is perfectly designed!

I am sure many of you with chronic conditions such as IBS or persistent headaches have noticed that you tend to experience increased pain levels when you force yourself to do something that you really don't want to do, such as giving a presentation at work, or when you are irritated by someone. This is because we are not the best at embracing our emotions. All too often, our response is to ignore, suppress, or override those uncomfortable feelings, and our brain's response is to cause pain in an attempt to get our attention. The brain interprets our fearful or anxious thoughts and suppressed emotions as dangerous. It is always doing its best to protect us and point us towards healing, even though it might not feel like it when we are experiencing pain.

Persisting Pain Overprotects Us and Prevents Recovery

The longer our pain persists, the more protective our system becomes because the brain senses permanent danger. This causes reduced range of motion, reduced activity levels, spreading pain, and increasing pain intensity. This overprotective system prevents us from giving the tissues what they need to recover and return to normal.

Imagine this scene: You are walking to the top of a tall cliff. Once you reach the top, a fence about one metre from the edge keeps you safe and prevents you from getting too close to the edge.

The fence is like 'pain' – protecting us from injury. When we are injured, the fence automatically moves further back from the cliff edge, and as we heal, it moves back towards the edge. In persistent pain, however, the fence moves further away from the cliff edge. This happens through a process called bioplasticity, which means an adaptive change in your biology.

This growing buffer area is our brain's attempt to keep us safe. The brain tends to overrule the body, preventing us from performing everyday activities that allow our tissues to heal. This overprotection is challenging because it weakens tissues and prevents normal healing.

The buffer becomes too big, and our world gets smaller and smaller as we lose movement and confidence and maybe even stop going out. Our pain system has become hypersensitive, causing us to feel like we are still injured.

Pain is a conversation between body and brain, but as in any conversation, sometimes there are misunderstandings. The brain thinks it is in control, so what starts as protection can take over, causing the nervous system to get stuck in a cycle of habitual protection, even when the threat has gone.

The good news is that our body has an irresistible force of healing, so even though we are experiencing pain, we are safe. We just need to tell our brain that we are sore, yes, but we are safe.

Many Factors Influence Pain

There is no one single thing that causes pain. Pain is a multifaceted, complex system.

The old, outdated view was that pain receptors in our body are stimulated, sending pain signals via the spinal cord to the brain, producing pain. This old belief that body parts alone produce pain is untrue.

Pain is NOT simply a signal that something is wrong in the body, but rather a protective response generated by our mind's response to perceived threats. In other words, thoughts and thinking can contribute to the experience of pain.

We've all heard stories or seen video clips of someone being able to save a loved one from a car wreck despite having two broken arms, or scoring a goal in a football game despite running on an obviously broken lower leg.

These people have suffered a traumatic injury but are not experiencing pain. Pain signals have not entered their consciousness, as they are not thinking about the injury. Their focus is on the task at hand, demonstrating that we only experience pain when it comes into our consciousness.

We need Mind, Consciousness, and Thought to experience anything in life, including pain.

> **Mind** refers to the life force powering our minds and our cells, something beyond ourselves. We see Mind when a cut on our finger heals from the inside out and when our body knows to take its next breath.

> **Consciousness** is awareness, how we focus on a thought and make it feel real to us.

> **Thought** is a psychological and spiritual gift that humans use to create their experience of life.

Our thoughts play a massive role in our pain experience and our body's ability to heal. When we struggle with persistent pain, we think about it – a lot! This is human and understandable. We might feel worried, frustrated, anxious, and fearful about what the pain means. We are, after all, thinking creatures; we have tens of thousands of thoughts every day. The problem is not that we have these thoughts. We can't control that, but by grabbing the thought and giving it our attention, it grows and, in turn, creates a whole new set of thoughts, causing us to get stuck in a story filled with fearful thinking that signals to our brains that we are in danger.

The opportunity here is to notice the thought and let it go.

> *"You cannot keep birds from flying over your head, but you can keep them from nesting in your hair."*
>
> Martin Luther (1483–1546)
>
> German priest, theologian, and author of the Explanation of the Lord's Prayer, Sixth Petition

The amount of attention we pay to a thought creates our experience in that moment. For example, if you walk past someone on the street you know and they appear to ignore you, you may think, "They must be upset with me; why are they ignoring me?" And if you give that thought some more attention and meaning, you will end up falling down a rabbit hole, consumed with a lot of thinking that will cause you to experience feelings of self-doubt. However, if at that moment you think, "They seemed very distracted; I do hope they're OK," then that thought is likely to generate feelings of concern and empathy instead.

Remember, it is not the events that happen in our lives that cause us to feel good or bad, but our interpretation of them.

Even perceiving a healthcare professional's comments as shaming or blaming can increase our experience of pain. Our thoughts don't have to be specifically about pain; they could be anxious thoughts about a stressful situation at work, a complicated relationship, or worrying about finances. The brain interprets these thoughts as a threat, and any such thoughts can easily trigger the already hypersensitive neural pathways in the brain that produce pain.

Research has shown that certain brain regions – the dorsal anterior cingulate cortext (dACC) and the anterior insula – are activated by both emotional distress and physical pain. A study in *Proceedings of the National Academy of Sciences* found that intense social rejection activates areas in the brain associated with the sensory components of physical pain, (Kross et al, 'Social rejection shares somatosensory representations with physical pain,' March 2011).

Additionally, research discussed in *Frontiers in Neuroscience* discusses how stress affects areas such as the prefrontal cortex, hippocampus, amygdala, and hypothalamus, which are all involved in processing physical pain, (Zheng et al, 'The Neurobiological Links between Stress and Traumatic Brain Injury,' August 2023). These findings all suggest that emotional pain often manifests in the same way as physical pain. I'm sure we have all heard someone describe the loss of a loved one as a physical ache in their heart.

When I tore a disc in my back four years ago and struggled with persistent pain 16 weeks later (even though the disc would have healed), I realised I was caught up in my thoughts, worrying about whether I would ever get back to work again, afraid that I was going to need surgery and upset that I was letting my patients down. I was stuck in a stress response and my brain was producing pain to save me from the perceived danger.

When my back was in spasm, I was also overtreating myself, doing exercises every few hours, determined to make myself better, but the harder I tried to get rid of the pain, the more I was reinforcing that the pain was dangerous.

It wasn't until I saw this and began to tell myself I was going to be OK, even if I did need surgery, that my pain suddenly began to reduce and resolve. I caught myself when I had a negative thought and refused to buy into it, lowering the danger level in my brain.

Less Danger Means Less Pain

All my fear and attention had been fuelling my pain. My thinking had turned on my threat physiology, perpetuating my body's inflammation and pain.

A more up-to-date understanding teaches us that pain is a danger alarm system, not just a tissue injury alarm system. Pain is our brain's opinion of danger, and that opinion does not always reflect reality.

Remember the builder who fell from scaffolding and landed on a six-inch nail? The nail had not even pierced his skin, yet he was experiencing pain. His pain was real; it was his brain's interpretation of this event as dangerous.

Understanding the Inside-Out Nature of Life

This section is vital as it helps us understand how our experience of life is created. Now that we better understand why we experience pain and how persistent pain arises, we must see the inside-out nature of our experience as human beings.

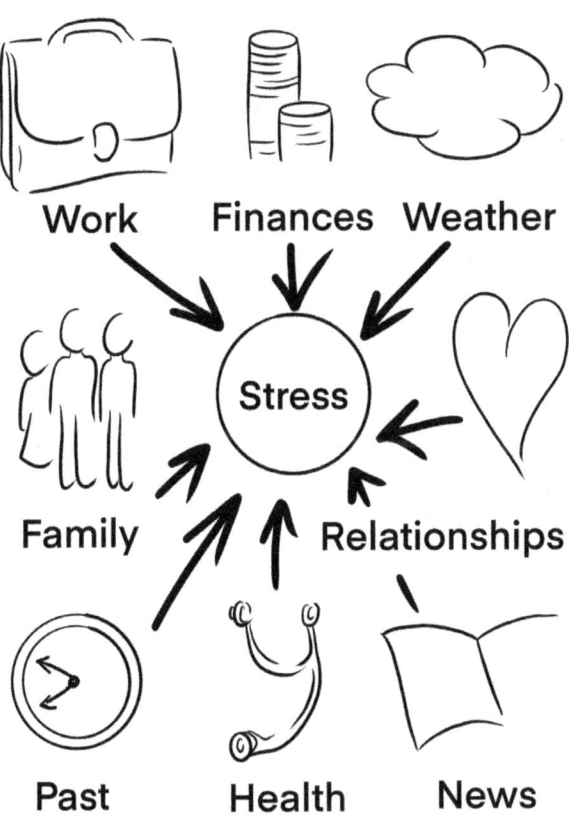

We tend to believe that circumstances, people, or situations outside of us make us feel a certain way, but I have news for you: it is the opposite! Life is an inside-out experience. Let me explain: If two people sustain the exact same injury, one might scream blue murder and complain about every bit of help offered while another copes well, grateful for the help and taking their discomfort in their stride. The difference is created by what is going on inside their heads: their thoughts.

We are all living in the feeling of our thoughts 100% of the time

If we happen to have one too many anxious thoughts about our pain, this can tip us into a stress response in our body. And if we are struggling with persistent pain, our pain pathways are already so hypersensitive that one thought might be enough to trigger those neural pathways in our brain, resulting in more pain. Once our system becomes hypersensitive (the fence has moved way back from the cliff edge, creating a bigger buffer), our initial injury has most likely healed itself, but we are still experiencing pain. Our fearful, frustrated, anxious, stressful thinking innocently perpetuates our pain.

Our pain loop is really a fear loop. We feel pain, and then we begin to worry about the pain; the pain gets worse, and so we fear the pain even more, which causes us to experience even more pain. It becomes a vicious circle, and it is difficult to break free.

We have all had anxious thoughts pop into our minds, and before we know it, we have innocently added lots more thinking on top of it and get caught up in a thought storm. We all experience this because our thoughts appear to be so true. But remember, it's just like a bad dream; when we wake up to the fact that it is a dream, we are relieved. What if we could wake up to the illusion that our thoughts are creating our experience and instead choose to paint a new picture?

What we pay attention to grows, so next time you think, "There's that flipping pain again," try not to attach other thoughts to it. Know that each thought will pass, just as clouds pass in the sky, and so too will the pain.

Creating safety rather than danger is the key to understanding persistent pain. So it's not about controlling or changing our thinking; it's just about recognising that we are innocently caught up in our thinking and trusting that it will pass.

When we step out of the thought storm into the space beyond thought, our body and mind experience more peace. We feel more at home and safe here. In other words, the quieter our mind, the quieter our body will become.

In closing, I want to share something powerful with you. Your feelings are an internal radar, telling you if you are caught up in a thought storm that might trigger your pain or symptoms.

All feelings, including emotions and sensations, are love letters from your body, guiding you back into balance. When you feel angry, afraid, depressed, frustrated, in pain, or anxious, it shows you that your thinking is 'off base' and not to be trusted.

Our body is never working against us; it is always working for us

We are not broken! Layers of thinking have simply covered over our innate health and well-being, thinking that we have innocently believed to be true.

Key Takeaways

◊ **Pain Protects and Promotes Healing:** Pain is the brain's interpretation of danger, aimed at protecting and promoting recovery.

◊ **Persistent Pain Overprotects and Prevents Recovery:** Chronic pain amplifies the protective mechanisms of the brain; overprotection perpetuates pain, and shrinks the individual's world.

◊ **Pain is Influenced by Multiple Factors:** Pain is not merely a physical signal but a complex, multifaceted experience – understanding and addressing this can reduce it.

◊ **The Inside-Out Nature of Life:** Our experience of pain is shaped by our thoughts and interpretations, not external circumstances.

Chapter 10

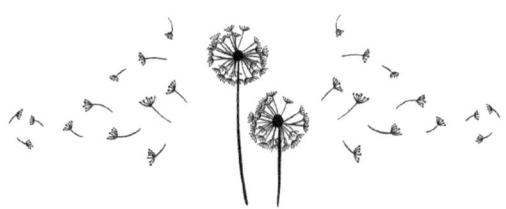

Words Create Our Reality

My Story

WHEN I WAS 12, I HATED *when my class timetable said it was time for English. My stomach would fill with butterflies, and I prayed my English teacher wouldn't pick on me. He often called me to the front of the class to read. My worst nightmare was reading aloud in front of the class. I got so nervous that I stuttered and stammered over the simplest words. The words did not make sense, and my face would grow redder and redder. One particular day, when his patience ran out, the teacher shouted, "Julie Doyle, you are dyslexic and illiterate and will amount to nothing!" in front of the whole class. I sincerely believed his words to be true. They became engrained in my head; keeping me quiet, shy, and insecure for most of my life – until I began to see that this belief was, in fact, just a thought.*

I'm pretty sure everyone reading this book has their own version of this story. Maybe it's time to ask yourself, "Is it completely true? Is it absolutely true, or is it a story I've made up with my thoughts and thinking about what was said to me?"

I now see that I innocently believed this story because of my thinking about it until about five years ago when I chose to let go of those thoughts and instead became a published author!

I share this story to emphasise the power of words. This is especially evident when we consider the placebo effect, an important phenomenon in healthcare that has been extensively documented. Numerous research studies unequivocally prove its existence.

These studies, with their intriguing design, feature a control group of subjects and a placebo group. In a fascinating twist, the control group receives the actual treatment, while the placebo group does not.

A placebo is a positive effect on health or symptoms that happens because of a person's belief in a treatment, even if the treatment itself has no active ingredients. A nocebo is a negative effect on health or symptoms that happens because of a person's expectation of harm, even if there is no actual harmful cause.

The key is that the placebo group is told they have a 50% chance of receiving a legitimate treatment that will help and a 50% chance of receiving something inert.

This phenomenon was observed in a 1983 study conducted by the British Stomach Cancer Group (Fielding et al, 1983). In this study, 411 participants were informed that nausea and hair loss were potential side effects of a new chemotherapy treatment. Remarkably, in the placebo group (which received only a benign substance), over 30% of participants experienced hair loss and 56% reported vomiting! This outcome highlights the significant impact of the *nocebo* effect, where negative expectations can lead to the manifestation of adverse symptoms, even in the absence of an active treatment.

So the placebo effect is when belief helps, and the nocebo effect is when belief harms.

Such is the power of suggestion and belief!

The Mind is a powerful creator; the thoughts we believe and the words we use determine our life experiences, including pain.

All too often, patients walk into my treatment room with a printout of their scan results. Even though they can't fully understand the medical jargon, they are very attached to their report. They focus on terms such as degenerative changes, wear and tear, bulging discs, or a tear in the annular wall of the disc. They believe the test results are a life sentence because they are printed in black-and-white print on a piece of paper, with their name and date of birth at the top.

Similarly, I have had many patients over the years who are very attached to the diagnosis they have received. Referring to "MY fibromyalgia" or "MY arthritis", their 'disorder' becomes their identity, while all along, they are more than their body or their diagnosis. Yes, they have been given a diagnosis of fibromyalgia, but it is not who they are.

A diagnosis is a marker of where you are in that moment, not who you are!

I recently heard Professor Peter O'Sullivan, a specialist Musculoskeletal Physiotherapist from Australia, discuss a study (yet to be published) in which patients with acute low back pain were scanned and divided into two groups. Everyone in the first group was told their scan results were typical for their age, with no cancer, fractures, or cause for concern. This first group were not given the details of their scan results, including disc bulges, degeneration, etc. The researchers told everyone in the second group about their scan results and they were given specific information about bulging discs, degenerative changes, bony spurs, etc. Subjects were, again, reassured that cancer and fractures had been ruled out.

On review two months later, everyone in the first group had improved, their pain was resolving, and movement/function was returning to normal. However, everyone in the second group continued to struggle with persistent pain along with a loss of mobility and function.

This shows how words and beliefs create our experience. There are many other studies showing how negative language in the healthcare setting increases anxiety levels, strengthens the experience of illness, and reduces treatment outcomes (Fieke Linskens et al., 2023).

Every time we say, "I'm stuck in this body," or "I'm never going to get better," or "My body is broken," we send these beliefs and thoughts about our illness to every cell in our body. Our mind and body are one. Each fearful thought we have about our diagnosis or pain hinders our body's natural ability to heal. We are innocently sending signals to the body that we are damaged.

Our thoughts create when we give them fuel! The more someone believes their negative thoughts about pain, the more their pain is exacerbated, which promotes feelings of stress and anxiety, helplessness and hopelessness, and even fear, resulting in social isolation and lack of movement.

Medical terminology can reinforce our hopelessness and helplessness and even cause catastrophising. The language we use will reinforce how we feel and how we experience our pain.

The placebo effect engages an innate capacity to heal. In other words, if we believe we are being given something that will aid our healing and recovery, it often engages the body's own healing capacity.

As a healthcare professional, I have become much more aware of my words when talking to my patients, especially when they ask me for my opinion about their diagnoses. The last thing I want to do is cause fear or label them with something that consumes their thinking and becomes their reality. So, instead, I point out how powerful and adaptive their body is, helping them take steps in a more healing, truthful direction.

Key Takeaways

◊ **The Power of Words and Beliefs:** Words and beliefs shape our experiences; negative words leave lasting psychological scars; positive beliefs enhance recovery.

◊ **Diagnosis vs. Identity:** A diagnosis reflects a moment in time, not a person's identity. Patients are often too attached to medical labels, when they are much more than their condition.

◊ **The Mind-Body Connection:** Thoughts and language influence physical well-being. The negative hinder our natural ability to heal, whilst the positive fosters resilience and recovery.

◊ **The Role of Healthcare Communication:** Healthcare professionals must use empowering and neutral language. Negative explanations about diagnoses can worsen patient outcomes.

Chapter 11

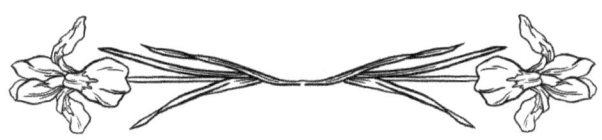

Soul's Wisdom

WE'VE ALL HEARD THE expression 'body, mind, and soul.' So far, we have discussed the body and the mind, but what about the soul?

I recently started to realise the importance of listening to my soul.

How often do we stop and ask our soul what it wants us to know? When I asked this of my soul, parts of this chapter were revealed.

Connecting with our soul can be a fantastic healing experience. It's often described as a feeling of pure bliss. When I connect with my soul, I feel joy, overwhelming gratitude, and peace. I feel connected, safe, and protected. These feelings are available, and bathing in them is where healing resides.

Here are some definitions of 'soul' from some top spiritual teachers:

"Your soul is the part of you that is always whole, even when everything else is falling apart."

Eckhart Tolle
Author of *The Power of Now* and a spiritual teacher known for his teachings on mindfulness

"The soul is the light of the body. When the soul is fully awakened, it shines through the eyes."

Paramahansa Yogananda
Hindu spiritual leader and author of *Autobiography of a Yogi*

"The soul is the essence of who you are, your true identity beyond the physical body."

Deepak Chopra
Prominent figure in the New Age movement, known for his writings on quantum physics and spirituality

Michael Singer, author of *The Untethered Soul*, refers to the soul as **the witness** – the unchanging awareness behind all thoughts, emotions, and experiences. He teaches that by detaching from the mind and allowing life to flow, we free the soul from limitations and experience profound peace.

Each of these definitions shares a common thread: the soul is not the body or mind but a deeper, limitless essence that connects us to something greater. Which definition resonates most with you?

Not just a philosophical concept, the soul is an integral part of humanity, deeper than our personality. Before our physical form, there is a spiritual essence to who we are, and our soul is a part of the whole spirit in each of us. It is defined as *"the spiritual or immaterial part of a human being"* (Collins English Dictionary). It is believed to continue to exist in some form even after the body has died.

So where does the soul come into the picture?

The soul is where wisdom resides. Just as our body communicates through 'feelings' such as sensations and emotions, so does our soul commune with us. Our soul communicates with us when we drop out of the noise of our personal thinking into the space beyond thought.

If this sounds complicated, let me put it another way. The soul communicates through stillness and moments of clarity, often arising when distractions are set aside. It happens most often to me when I am walking the dogs. It's not intentional, but as I walk through the forest, I look at the tall oak trees and am amazed by their strength and beauty. I am fascinated by the moss continuing to grow on the fallen branches, and before I know it, something new pops into my mind – a thought, an idea that brings clarity and sometimes even creativity. Clarity or insight never arises when I'm caught up in a lot of busy thinking, the noise so loud that I don't even notice the robin sitting on top of the waste bin as I walk close by!

Humans have developed some terrible habits. Endless scrolling on our phones is just one habit that distracts us from being more present. We ignore our bodies as they try to get our attention, and we forget to commune with our souls. I must confess: I've been guilty of the above.

Even after working as a physiotherapist for over 35 years, it wasn't until around eight years ago that I discovered the importance of listening to my body. Before this, I believed that pain, sensations, or emotions were simply signs that something was broken and needed to be fixed.

When we have pain, we look to the physical for healing, but what if we included something more profound and available to us all: our soul?

Our soul is always pointing us towards health and well-being, but our humanness tends to block out the voice of our soul. As our humanness grapples for control, it takes over at the expense of our body and soul. But we are body, mind, and soul, so we need to pay attention to all of us. When we ignore a part of who we are, dis-ease can take root in the system. Being present to all that is allows wisdom to flow and innate well-being to flourish.

Although we often refer to our soul as being in a higher consciousness, it is right here within us. Our soul has infinite wisdom and knowledge to share with us, and it desires to communicate, connect and bring wisdom, pointing us towards healing and wholeness.

I have recently started a simple practice of taking three deep breaths and asking my soul what it wants me to know. Then, I begin to write automatically. What ends up on the page is truly incredible. The words are steeped in love, which can be felt at a cellular level. It's like connecting with your best friend, who you haven't seen in years.

Regarding the experience I shared at the start of this book, where I struggled with constant pain for over 18 weeks after injuring my back, it wasn't until my mind became quiet after reading the poem that a new thought popped up about detaching from the outcome. This realisation resulted in letting go of all the striving to fix myself, which, in turn, allowed my body to heal.

In *The Missing Link*, Sydney Banks states, *"When the wise tell us to look within, they are directing us beyond intellectual analysis of personal thought to a higher order of knowledge called wisdom. Wisdom is an innate intelligence everyone possesses deep within their souls, before the contamination of the outer world of creation."*

Our body's ability to heal is connected to how we use our personal mind, but the whispers of our soul also play a crucial role. The soul's wisdom is always available to us when we allow our minds to settle. Wisdom connects us not only to healing but also to something greater – the interconnected nature of life itself.

When we access the wisdom of the soul, we begin to see that healing is not just an individual process – it is deeply connected to the fabric of life itself. Just as we cannot separate a wave from the ocean, we cannot separate ourselves from the greater intelligence of the universe. Our souls are intimately connected to a manifestation of something bigger than us. We are not just a body, a mind, or a soul in isolation – we are part of a much larger whole. We are the energy of Universal Mind, and we never lose that connection to something greater than us.

Interconnectedness

I don't know about you, but I used to think I was my body and anything that was not my body or me was outside of me or separate from me. However, through the gift of the Three Principles, I have experienced the oneness of all that is. We are not separate.

We can now see that we use the gifts of Mind, Thought, and Consciousness to create our experience of life. So, if thoughts create, why do we often hold onto and feed painful memories, uncomfortable thoughts, hurts, insecurities, anxieties, and negative feelings? We constantly forget there is a choice – to connect with the wisdom of our soul and experience feelings of peace and joy instead.

When we hang out in thoughts of suffering and pain, the attention we give this thinking only serves to incorrectly confirm to our brain and nervous system that we are in danger and that we need protection.

It is simple! Our personal thinking feeds the threat that our body feels and keeps it alive.

Of course, tragic and traumatic events happen in life, leaving us feeling powerless. Sometimes, we heal quickly, accepting our pain, finding perspective, and moving on, but sometimes, we heal slowly. Healing has its own timing and can often be slower than we want. The mystery of timing is the soul's wisdom.

I could share many examples from my life of slowly healing or struggling to heal because I got so caught up in my thinking. The story I told myself became so loud that I was deafened to the wisdom inside.

One of my mentors, Deborah Epstein, says, *"Healing is a journey, an unfolding of the truth of who we really are. It is a journey through the holding, bracing, and belief patterns in the bodymind. As they unravel, the pain eases. Healing is a catalyst for the change our soul wants us to make. We all come to our truth in our own time and in our own way. We are body, mind, and soul, a multidimensional web of wonder and creative life force."* (https://deborahepstein.substack.com/p/transform-fear-into-freedom-the-power)

When we come into oneness, unity, and love – into Divine consciousness – it's here that we find unconditional love for ourselves. It's here that we come to know ourselves beyond doubt, pain, wounds, fear, and anxiety, to know ourselves as we have never known ourselves before – as whole, complete, and loved.

*"No matter which path you take, the wisdom you seek will always be found within the depths of your **own** consciousness."*

Sydney Banks
The Missing Link

When we experience chronic pain, it's easy to feel disconnected – from our bodies, from hope, and even from life itself. We often search for external solutions, looking for something outside of us to "fix" the pain. But what if healing also involves something deeper? Our soul's wisdom is always guiding us towards wholeness, yet when we are caught in cycles of stress, fear, and resistance, we can't hear its gentle whispers. By quieting the mind and reconnecting with the deeper essence of who we are, we open the door to profound healing. Just as my moment of insight allowed me to let go and, in turn, created space for my body to heal, we can all access this wisdom when we shift our focus from striving and struggling to stillness and trust. Healing isn't just about the body – it's an unfolding of the whole self, a return to the truth of who we really are.

Healing is always possible, and it can happen slowly or rapidly. Bruises heal, broken bones heal, wounds heal. Healing is at its best when we follow our soul's wisdom.

Soul's Quest

As I listen to my body,
something cracks open deep inside.
I hear my soul.

As I rediscover my body,
feeling safe enough to climb back inside
I touch my essence.

She is soft; she is tender.
She moves like liquid
when I let go.

All along she has been hiding under the surface
dwelling in the shallow waters of my being.

She longs to be held gently in my heart.
Love is her language.
Always available when I ask for help.
She swaddles me in unconditional love.

Pure and wise, she lives in my greatest depth.
I have the power to call her into form.

She is present.
She serves.
She heals.
She replenishes and restores.
She is love.

As I learn to drop inside,
I feel rooted in her presence.
Her softness can be felt in my breath.

When I rest, I can feel her peace.
Each time I return,
She sets me free.

Choosing to stop tightening and bracing against life,
I have found her comforting touch.

As I learn to speak a new language to my body,
One of well-being,
One of restoration,
One of grace.

I am breathing the soft one within me awake.
As I listen to her message,
I am learning to listen to my soul.

From my book, Finding Mystery Within

Key Takeaways

◊ **The Soul as a Source of Wisdom and Healing:** The soul is ever-present within us, distinct from body and mind. It communicates via insight, leading to clarity, creativity, and healing.

◊ **The Importance of Listening to the Soul:** Ignoring the soul creates imbalance and dis-ease, while using simple practices to tune into its wisdom fosters peace and well-being.

◊ **Thoughts Shape Our Experience:** Pain and suffering stem from the thoughts we focus on. By focusing on the wisdom of the soul, we create space for healing and transformation.

◊ **The Interconnection of Body, Mind, and Soul:** When we embrace our wholeness – body, mind, and soul – this leads us to being connected to something greater than ourselves.

Chapter 12

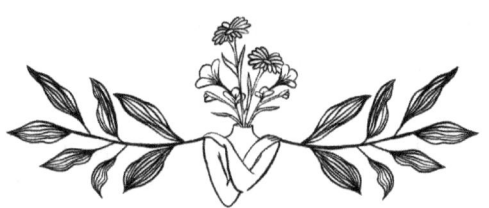

Harnessing the Wisdom of Your Body

WE ALL TEND TO RESIDE in our heads/personal minds, with our thoughts consuming us. In other words, we live from the neck up, ignoring our bodies unless they are clever enough to gain our attention somehow. We each have the gift of a shimmering awareness that lies deep within our bodies, but we all too often ignore it. The body communicates through sensations, such as pain, tightness, tension, discomfort, or emotions, such as anger, fear, or anxiety, as well as the good ones, such as joy, peace, or lightness. Every feeling and emotion belongs, not just the good ones. Our body communicates this way to show us if we are on the right path.

Now I understand what Sydney Banks meant when he repeatedly said, *"Follow the feeling, look for the nice feeling."*

(*Hawaii lecture series*). In other words, the not-so-nice feelings simply show us that our thinking has veered off course.

Feelings, whether sensations or emotions, are an integral part of our lives. They connect us to the reality we experience and mirror our current mental state, indicating whether our thoughts are beneficial or harmful.

The body holds the key; after all, feelings reside here. I am learning the importance of simply noticing what I am feeling with love and curiosity instead of acting on them (possibly destructively) or harbouring, denying or repressing them. It's common to label certain feelings as harmful or unwanted. However, emotions like anger, fear, anxiety, or pain are not to be fought against or ignored. They are part of our innate wisdom, trying to communicate with us. We must not fear our feelings; they are our guide and whispers of wisdom.

I've seen that when we ignore or mask the not-so-nice feelings, the body usually shouts louder. I see this daily when taking a patient's history. They will share how their symptoms started, and when they ignored them or did nothing about it, their symptoms intensified or spread to other areas of their body. I've also seen this time and time again in my own life.

Love Letters

Dr Bill Pettit refers to our feelings as "love letters" in disguise, each feeling guiding us towards health and healing. I think this is beautiful.

I have also heard Dr Pettit explain that one of three things will happen when we innocently grab hold of anxious thoughts and give them our attention.

1. Our anxiety levels increase.

2. Our mood goes down.

3. Our body starts to hurt somewhere.

I know from experience that more than one of these can co-occur.

Each of us has innate health inside; it gets covered over and held captive by layers of our thinking, causing us to forget it exists as our body screams out, trying to get our attention. It makes sense that the body's healing intelligence is released by love, peace, and acceptance; these feelings bring us home to a place of contentment, where we live a rich, satisfying life in the moment, whether we physically heal or not.

There is no predicting where or how physical healing will manifest in our bodies. However, science supports this belief in innate health by showing that when we bathe our cells in more healing substances called neuropeptides – molecules of emotions, such as acceptance, faith or understanding – healing will express itself through our cellular wisdom. This is the infinite potential of Mind playing out in our body as seen in the work of Dr Candace Pert, such as *Molecules of Emotion*.

The mind and body are not separate but part of a seamless, intricate intelligence network. I am constantly blown away by just how amazing the body is! We all have a fascial web that surrounds every single cell in our body and weaves us together into physical form so our soul can live on earth. This web is the container of our consciousness, through which divine intelligence flows and takes form as thoughts, our ability to think.

> *"We each are in charge of how we see, feel and think about the world. And because we create from our senses, deep within our body, the health and well-being of the bodymind complex is in our hands."*
>
> Deborah Epstein

I now understand that life is not happening to us; it is happening through us. We participate in this journey by being conscious of the thoughts that give us our life experiences. Our body responds instantly to our thoughts, and if we know that fear, anxiety, depression, anger, and grief are all destructive to our physical health, we learn to allow these emotions to wash freely over us rather than resisting or fearing them. We trust that without our attention and judgement, they will pass through without a ripple, allowing the healing energy in us to flow unimpeded.

Acceptance of our humanity frees us from the burden of chronic stress and self-judgement. It prevents these negative emotions from accumulating at a cellular level and wreaking havoc on our bodies.

During a personal crisis, I remember a conversation with my coach, Dr Linda Sandel Pettit, when I struggled with some very sticky thoughts that felt real. These thoughts repeatedly played in my head, and I just could not get past them. I knew that I was tormenting myself. I was living in the experience of my thinking, but I just could not get past it. Knowing that my feelings were inseparable from thought, I was full of self-judgement, thinking, *"I should know better."*

However, Linda told me it was OK to make space for my feelings and let them flow through, not to judge myself or try to work things out. She gave me permission to be gentle with myself, and I began to see that I could make space and hold each emotion with compassion. Then she said, **"Let thoughts go and feelings be."**

This line struck a chord; it felt like I could suddenly give up the struggle. Then, I dropped the judgement and accepted my humanity; I let go of a lot of thinking, sat with my feelings and found peace in my body.

By discovering how our experience, whether happy or sad, is created from Mind, Consciousness, and Thought, we can find a way out of our suffering.

A body whose wisdom has never been honoured does not easily trust. We must learn to listen to our bodies and be responsible for knowing and loving them. Long before you do, your body knows when something is wrong. The clue is in the feelings or sensations it produces. Something is off when we feel tightness, tension, and anxiety. On the other hand, we also know that if something resonates in our body, we feel it in our gut as softness, calm, or ease.

When thoughts become embedded in our consciousness, they also become embedded in our body because consciousness is a full-body experience. As I deepen my understanding of how much power my thoughts have over my body, I am slowly letting go of so many old beliefs and judgements about myself that I've innocently held onto for far too long. I am a 'work in progress'! There are always a few sticky thoughts that I struggle to believe are just thoughts, and there always will be, as I'm human, after all. But when I have a moment of clarity, I see that a particular thought is not true, and my grip slowly and naturally releases.

When our thinking changes, our consciousness and experience change. Our levels of consciousness change with our thinking as we see the world through a different 'thought' lens. Only if someone's thinking shifts on its own can they change from the inside. When our thinking changes, we will change; if it doesn't, we won't.

> *"Once such knowledge has been seen,*
> *change in both the mind and body often occur."*
>
> Sydney Banks
> *In Quest of the Pearl*

Love, Acceptance and Compassion

The power of Thought is the bridge between the formless mind, which powers the brain, and the form, the body. When a thought arises and enters our awareness, a feeling accompanies that thought. The feeling occurs simultaneously, and we have no control over what arises. The more we see this is how life works, the less judgement we tend to have of ourselves.

However, if our thoughts and hearts lack love, we will live in a distressed and imbalanced body. But if our hearts are filled with love, thoughts will build strength, health and balance.

Love helps guide us through life, keeping us in harmony with our bodies, nature, and fellow human beings. What would it be like to honour each physical experience that arises in our body, turn towards it, commune with it, and listen to our body's intelligence?

We have discussed how the noise of our thoughts can be overwhelming, especially when we find ourselves stuck in a cycle of thoughts about our pain. These feelings of overwhelm can cause us to get lost in our symptoms. From here, we can return to the space beyond our thoughts, where well-being and clarity reside.

I love the image of a snow globe after it has just been shaken (from Chapter 5); the snowflakes represent our hundreds of thoughts, and it becomes difficult to see what sits inside. But as the snowflakes (thoughts) settle, we can see more clearly.

When we innocently get caught up in our thought-created reality, we block out the wisdom we need. Our humanness causes us to become deaf to subtle whispers of wisdom, so we often choose to ignore them. But as we learn to listen to the guiding power of wisdom, we begin to see that it empowers our body and soul, reconnecting us with the limitless Mind.

Discovering an innate internal compass that guides us with insights from a deeper, wiser source than ourselves is incredible.

Remember that feelings are love letters. So, accepting our emotions or sensations is critical, even when they might feel uncomfortable. Remember that they help us navigate life, like our very own inbuilt GPS, guiding us back home. When we let go of thoughts, we sink back into the quiet space where we can harness our body's wisdom, which calls us home into presence and peace.

When we see pain as an invitation to stop and be silent, often, the 'thoughts' we are listening to that are not true are revealed. Then, it's simply a matter of letting go of those thoughts instead of trying to think our way out of the pain. Allowing the snowflakes to settle brings clarity and freedom from the struggle.

Key Takeaways

◊ **The Body as a Messenger:** Emotions and physical sensations are the body's way of communicating. Pain or anxiety are "love letters" that carry wisdom, urging us to listen.

◊ **Mind-Body Connection:** Thoughts directly influence physical health. Conscious awareness of thoughts and feelings can help release stress and foster well-being.

◊ **Acceptance and Compassion:** Embrace emotions with curiosity and kindness, rather than judgement or repression, allows healing to unfold naturally.

◊ **Inner Compass of Wisdom:** By letting go of intrusive thoughts and connecting with our inner wisdom, we return to a state of balance and harmony.

Chapter 13

Our Guide Inside

SOMETIMES, WHEN WE feel stuck in a body we've been told is broken, our symptoms consume us. We live from a place where everything becomes about our bodies. But we are more than our bodies! We are an expression of Mind, Consciousness, and Thought; we are souls in motion.

On your journey through this book, you have seen how you can align with Mind, Consciousness, and Thought to heal your body, empowering yourself along the way and bringing a deeper connection to your soul.

The ultimate answers to all our struggles come from a realisation of the spiritual wisdom we already have inside, rather than constantly searching for information, treatments, and solutions outside. (Hear me when I say wisdom might point us towards something, as it did for me when I came across Myofascial Release on my healing journey from chronic fatigue/fibromyalgia labels.) But placing all our trust and hope in something out there often ends in disappointment. We can't look to something outside of us to change how we feel inside, but that doesn't stop us from trying.

> "...look within because the vastness of the physical earth and sky with all its solar systems is miniscule compared to what lies within every living soul walking the face of this earth."
>
> Sydney Banks,
>
> *The Missing Link*

Not only are we part of the intelligence behind the universe, but that intelligence or 'wisdom' is also within us. We are all guided through life, and this intelligence is always on our side; it always has our back. Symptoms are not something going wrong; they are simply divine intelligence trying to get our attention. They invite us not to panic but to listen and trust that our body has an innate capacity to heal. All of life is conspiring to heal us.

What if a disease is the cure in progress? So often, we resist, fight against and look for a quick fix outside through someone or something. We view symptoms as the enemy. But what if we befriend them, get into the right relationship with them and rather than trying to get rid of the dis-ease, find a place of ease with them and allow healing to come? What if we choose to allow the flow of life to carry us, knowing what we resist persists?

When I hurt my back in 2019, I spent over 18 weeks striving, pushing, ignoring my body and attempting to fix myself. I did not need surgery, I was not broken, and I did not need to be fixed; I just needed to listen to my body as it guided me back home. I needed to learn how to trust my guide inside as my soul helped me see that I was sore but safe.

The Isness

Last night, I listened to a guided meditation by Jamaican spiritual teacher Mooji called *An Invitation to Freedom* (see *Further Reading and Resources* for link). He talked about the isness/awareness that always is. If you've never heard the term 'the isness', and it sounds odd, we're in the same club. When I first heard it, I wondered what it was. But as I listened to Mooji's voice guiding me, I began to see that isness is when everything else falls away. It's a place where I have no thoughts, judgements, or ideas. I am fully present with my soul in the silence. There is no separation between me and what is as I sit in the isness. From this place, I am seeing more deeply that I am complete. Even though this was new to me, I could feel the embrace of love and peace. It felt like I was coming home into my body, and there was no separation between the isness and myself. I was immersed in the present moment, and it felt truly beautiful.

It's like that moment when the beauty of what you are looking at hits you; for example, when your firstborn baby comes into the world, all the pain and effort fade into a distant memory. An ocean wave crashes against the rocks as the sun sets in the background, and if you are fully present in the beauty of the scene in front of you, your worries disappear. So, for me, the isness refers to a spiritual sense that there is no separation between me and the healing energy behind life.

When we experience the isness, it may be the first time in a very long time, as we are so used to spending most of our time listening to the noise inside our heads. It feels like a homecoming. We will feel love seeping into every cell, and we will feel complete.

Love gives us the common sense, wisdom, and insights to deal with life and helps our bodies heal. Love, joy, and contentment live within. Remember that love is our default setting that gets obscured by layers of our thinking that we innocently believe to be true.

We **all** have access to this space beyond thought.

Our soul speaks directly to us, drawing us back into our bodies to a place of connection and oneness. Our soul tries to get our attention, showing us the answer to our suffering. Remember that when we use the gift of Thought as it was meant, we will find our way back to health and well-being.

Place your hand on your heart, and as you read these final lines, I pray you feel a connection, joy, and completeness you may never have felt before.

*Place a hand on your heart and take three deep breaths,
as you drop out of your head and into your body.*

Listen to the quiet…

*Travel deep inside your body, the seat of your soul,
In the stillness, allow your spinning thoughts to slow down.
In the silence, trust you are going to be OK,
In the peace, there is a knowing that things have a way of working out.*

*Stay present in this vessel that has carried you since you took your first breath,
Ever since your soul has been waiting for you to let it be your friend.
Telling you that everything you ever need is everything you are.*

*Feel free to ask your questions; your body holds the truth.
Even when your heart is heavy, and wounds have left their mark.
Remember, your soul was with you every place you've ever been.
It's the One that held you when you couldn't stand.
If you're wondering who can heal you, you can.*

*Your soul will meet you in the stillness.
Right here in your body, no need to look outside.
Always guiding you along the right path.
Have courage; your body and soul will show you how to listen, soften and heal.*

One of life's greatest gifts is the ability to return to a place of quiet and healing.

In a Quiet Mind, we are free of noise. Healing has lived in this state since the beginning of time. It's here that we learn to love and embrace our Quiet Body.

Key Takeaways

◊ **Inner Wisdom and Healing:** Trust the divine intelligence within to lead you towards healing and wholeness. Symptoms are signals guiding you back to balance and alignment.

◊ **Letting Go of Resistance:** Embrace your struggles with acceptance and ease rather than fighting against them. Trust and surrender will allow the flow of life to carry you towards healing.

◊ **Experiencing Isness:** Isness is a state of pure presence in which thoughts and judgements fall away. This connection to our soul fosters a sense of completeness and peace.

◊ **Returning to the Quiet:** In stillness and silence, your soul communicates with you, offering clarity and healing. A quiet mind and body allow you to reconnect with your essence.

Chapter 14

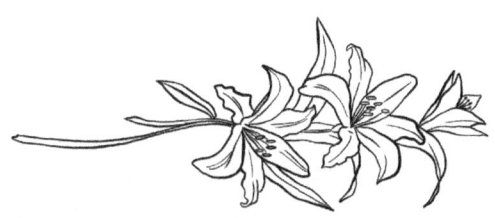

Mercy and Tenderness Heals

AS YOU APPROACH THE end of my book, I invite you to hear something even more profound. Over the last few years, this understanding of how the mind and body work together has slowly been seeping into my bones.

You are divine energy in form. You are Mind, God, Love, Wisdom, or Spirit, whatever you prefer. You are formless energy in motion.

Spiritual consciousness moves through you in the form of Thought, creating your life experience here on earth. You get to choose what you create.

I hear you say, *"But I hate my constant ill health; I'm never going to get better,"* or *" I'm so fed up with my pain; I'm useless; I can't even walk the dog."*

I hear you and want to tell you that this harsh inner dialogue often leads to more harm than good. It can leave scars as the harsh thoughts reinforce fear and anxiety. As you internalise these thoughts, they become hard-to-shake beliefs. All these judgements and thoughts, whether visible or invisible, become locked in the body.

But what would happen if you began to love that part of yourself? What if you learned to love yourself with your symptoms? What if you started to nurture yourself with compassion and kindness instead of judging yourself for not being perfect?

Don't fight against what your body is trying to do; instead, embrace and acknowledge it. Don't beat yourself up because you happen to believe something is broken. You are human. There is never going to be perfection in the form. Love yourself as you are, not when you overcome something. Love yourself so deeply that 'you' disappear. This has been a massive part of my healing journey; as I have let go of the need to control and fix my physical body, I have found myself in a place of coming home to the essence of who I am. I am a spiritual being in physical form, and the more time I spend nurturing and connecting with my essence, the more I am aware that I am already whole and complete.

Find compassion for yourself right now, including your pain, your anxiety, or your depression. Don't wait until you conquer it. Encourage yourself from a place of gentleness, understanding and deep self-acceptance. I'm not suggesting that you ignore your challenges or struggles, but I simply invite you to acknowledge them with kindness from a place of love. When you replace self-criticism and frustration with love and understanding, you will fall into the flow of life and stop fighting against what is. Small shifts can lead to profound changes. Leading with love will open up new possibilities and build resilience, confidence and a more profound sense of inner peace as you continue to heal, grow and evolve.

Take a breath, pause, and stop fighting and resisting your pain. Trust that your inner well of wisdom is bubbling up. Surrender to the flow.

Your human design is perfect, allowing divine intelligence to communicate with you, guiding you away from harm towards wholeness. It uses many different signals of expression to gain your attention, from physical symptoms to a low state of mind. When you ignore an ache in one part of your body, your body's intelligence might shift to a bout of vertigo to get your attention. It might be an emotion, a feeling, a physical symptom like pain, a memory or an insight. But whatever it is, it is simply your bodymind trying to get your attention to show you are heading off track: that you have separated from Love. Wisdom is calling; if you ignore it, it simply changes the channel.

All of life conspires to support your healing. Trust that there is a contagious force pulling you towards health and wholeness. Just as words create, so do beliefs. What if you could influence every single cell in your body in a different, healthier direction simply by the words you use when speaking about your body, health, or disease?

I pray you are open to finding out. Sit in this liminal space of 'not knowing' and wait for something new to unfold. All you have to do is respect and honour the divine intelligence behind your symptoms, viewing it as a key to open the door to where you need to go next.

This is a paradigm shift for many, but new possibilities will open up if you are open to seeing things differently. When you no longer fear your feelings, they become your guide, your whispers of wisdom, allowing you to feel your way into your healing.

Remember, you are loved, you are loving, you are lovable, always!

Key Takeaways

◊ **Embrace Your Divinity and Humanity:** You are divine energy in physical form, with the power to create your life experience.

◊ **Self-Love and Healing:** Replacing self-criticism with kindness transforms your healing journey. This shift fosters resilience, confidence, and peace.

◊ **Listening to Your Bodymind:** Symptoms, emotions, and physical sensations are signals from your inner wisdom, guiding you towards wholeness. Respect these messages as they hold the key to deeper healing.

◊ **The Power of Perspective and Belief:** By aligning with love and openness, you influence your body positively and allow new possibilities for growth and healing to emerge.

Appendices

Journaling Questions

HERE ARE SOME QUESTIONS designed to help you explore the connection between your thoughts, emotions, and physical pain. These aim to encourage reflection and foster insights. Jot your answers down in your journal or notebook.

Exploring Awareness and Pain

1. Have you noticed moments when you're so engaged in something that you forget about your pain? What were you doing in those moments?

2. When you focus on your pain, how does it feel compared to when your mind is occupied with something else?

3. What happens to your pain when you're completely relaxed or enjoying yourself?

Linking Stress and Pain

4. Have you observed a connection between times of stress or worry and the intensity of your pain?

5. When your thoughts are racing or filled with worry, how does your body respond?

6. Can you recall a time when you felt at peace, even if your pain was present? What was different about your thinking in that moment?

Understanding the Nature of Thoughts

7. What happens when you question the thoughts that arise about your pain? For example, "What if this pain doesn't mean what I think it means?"

8. How often do you notice yourself predicting or fearing the worst about your pain? How does that make you feel physically and emotionally?

9. If your pain could talk, what story would it be telling you? Do you believe that story is always true?

Shifting Perspective

10. How might your experience of pain change if you approached it with curiosity rather than resistance?

11. What if the thoughts about what your pain means or prevents you from doing are just thoughts? How might that shift your relationship with the pain?

12. If you didn't label your sensation as pain and just observed it, how would you describe what you feel?

Encouraging Empowerment

13. Have you ever noticed a small action or mindset shift that made your pain more manageable? What was it?

14. What's one thing you can do today, even if the pain is present, to remind yourself that you're more than your pain?

15. If you believed that your pain doesn't define you, what might become possible for you?

These questions gently encourage self-inquiry and create space for you to see the role of your thinking in perpetuating or easing your pain.

Glossary of Terms

Myofascial Release Therapy (MFR): A whole body treatment that addresses the fascial system in the body. It is a hands-on treatment that helps to bring the client out of their head and into their body, where they can become aware of places they are bracing or holding tension deep inside. Gentle sustained stretches/pressure is applied; the system is never forced.

Biopsychospiritual: A new model proposed by Julie McCammon to explain the many facets of chronic pain. Bringing the mind, body and soul into the frame.

Nociplastic pain: A type of ongoing pain that comes from changes in how the brain and nervous system process pain signals. It doesn't usually show up on scans or have a clear physical cause. The pain tends to move around the body, feels spread out, and people often struggle to point to exactly where it hurts.

Smudging: This occurs when the brain's map of the body gets a bit 'blurry' or confused. Normally, your brain knows exactly where each part of your body is and what it is feeling. But with ongoing pain, that map can become less clear – kind of like a smudged fingerprint. This can make pain feel stronger, harder to pinpoint, or even spread to nearby areas.

Crosstalk: This happens when different nerves or systems in the body start 'talking over' or interfering with each other, rather like when two phone lines get crossed. In the body, this can mean that signals from one area (like pain, stress, or tension) spill over and affect another area – even if that other part isn't injured or damaged. So, one part of the body might start hurting or reacting because it's 'picking up the noise' from somewhere else – not because something is wrong with it directly.

Neuroplasticity: The brain has the ability to change, adapt, and rewire itself – like flexible clay that can be reshaped. This means that the way we think, feel, and even experience pain can change over time, because the brain is always learning and forming new connections. It's how we form habits, learn new skills – and also how we can *unlearn* unhelpful patterns, like chronic pain or anxiety.

Adverse Childhood Experiences (ACEs): These are stressful or traumatic events that happen during childhood, such as abuse, neglect, or growing up in a home with violence, addiction, or mental illness. Research shows that having several ACEs can affect how the body and brain develop, and can increase the risk of health problems later in life – including chronic pain, anxiety, and heart disease.

Bioplasticity: This means that the body – just like the brain – has the ability to change and adapt over time. It refers to how our nervous system, muscles, tissues, and even pain responses can shift depending on things like movement, stress, injury, or even our thoughts and emotions. So if something in the body has changed in an unhelpful way (such as becoming overly sensitive or stiff), it also has the capacity to change back – to heal, adapt, and become more balanced again. Rather as a plant will lean towards the light, the body can 'lean' towards health when given the right conditions.

Further Reading and Resources

Foreword

People:

www.drbillpettit.com

Dr William (Bill) F. Pettit, Jr., M.D. is a board-certified psychiatrist and co-owner of 3 Principles Intervention LLC, dedicated to promoting mental well-being. Since 1983, he has been an international educator on the Three Universal Principles of Mind, Consciousness, and Thought. After retiring from clinical psychiatry in December 2018, he resumed practice in July 2024, offering telehealth services in Adrian, Michigan. In addition to his clinical work, Dr Pettit serves as an adjunct faculty member at Creighton University School of Medicine, where he supports medical students and contributes to the Diversity, Inclusion & Belonging

Committee. Dr Pettit is a faculty of American Holistic Nursing and his programs are eligible for CEUs from the California Nurse Association. Dr Pettit recently joined Hive Health Systems Limited as a Well-Being Consultant.

Dr Pettit's extensive educational background includes degrees from the University of Illinois College of Medicine and experiences as a U.S. Naval Flight Surgeon and Chief of Psychiatry at the U.S. Navy Nuclear Submarine Base. He has published numerous academic contributions and developed online courses to share his insights. Looking ahead, he is planning two legacy courses for 2025-2026, focused on innovative mental health paradigms and new understandings within psychiatry.

Introduction

People:

Dr Linda Sandel Pettit: www.lindasandelpettit.com

Ian Watson: www.theinsightspace.com

Chapter 1

Books:

McCammon, J, *Finding Mystery Within*, July 2021

Miller, L, *The Awakened Brain*, Penguin, 2022

People:

Sydney Banks: www.sydneybanks.org

Chapter 2

People:

Descartes, R, *Treatise of Man (Traite de l'homme)*, written 1633 but published posthumously 1644

Studies:

Melzack, R. & Wall, P.D. (November 1965). 'Pain mechanisms: a new theory' [PDF]. *Science*, 150(3699), 971–979. Bibcode: 1965Sci...150..971M. https://doi.org/10.1126/science.150.3699.971. PMID: 5320816. Archived from the original (PDF) on 14 January 2012.

Chapter 3

Books:

Sarno, J, *Healing Back Pain*, Warner Books, 1991

Sarno, J, *The Mindbody Prescription*, Little, Brown and Company, 1999

Sarno, J, *The Divided Mind*, Harper Collins, 2006

People:

Dr Howard Schubiner: www.unlearnyourpain.com

Dr Lorimer Moseley: www.tamethebeast.org

Chapter 4

Books:

Pert, C, *Molecules of Emotion*, Simon & Schuster, 1999

Banks, S, *The Missing Link*, Lone Pine Publishing, 1998

Chapter 5

People:

John F Barnes: www.myofascialrelease.com

Mavis Karn: www.maviskarn.net

Books:

Kelly, T.M., *Upside-Down and Backwards*, Reflections Counseling Center, 2022

Chapter 6

Podcast:

Your Life but Easier with Paola Royal: https://creators.spotify.com/pod/profile/yourlifebuteasier/episodes/Body-and-universal-Mind-Connection-e2uvv42

Chapter 7

Books:

Goswami, A, *The Self-Aware Universe*, Jeremy P Tarcher, 1993

Braden, G, *The Divine Matrix*, Hay House, 2007

Miller, L, *The Awakened Brain*, Penguin, 2022

Chopra, D, *Quantum Healing: Exploring the Frontiers of Mind/Body Medicine*, New Age, 1989

Chapter 8

Podcast:

Feel Better, Live More with Dr Rangan Chatterjee, Episode 310: www.drchatterjee.com/how-to-heal-chronic-pain-with-dr-howard-schubiner-re-release/

TEDx Talk:

Dr Lorimer Moseley, 'Why Things Hurt'
www.youtube.com/watch?v=gwd-wLdIHjs&list=PLeMJSyOw8AcVwJH1f9Q9qblnUpD32EPFJ&index=1

Books:

Banks, S, *The Enlightened Gardener*, Lone Pine Publishing, 2016

Chapter 9

Studies:

Kross, E., Berman, M.G., Mischel, W., Smith, E.E. & Wager, T.D. (2011). 'Social rejection shares somatosensory representations with physical pain.' *Proceedings of the National Academy of Sciences of the United States of America*, 108(15), 6270–6275. https://doi.org/10.1073/pnas.1102693108. Epub 28 March 2011. PMID: 21444827; PMCID: PMC3076808.

Zheng, L., Pang, Q., Xu, H., Guo, H., Liu, R. & Wang, T. (2022). 'The neurobiological links between stress and traumatic brain injury: a review of research to date.' *International Journal of Molecular Sciences*, 23(17), 9519. https://doi.org/10.3390/ijms23179519. PMID: 36076917; PMCID: PMC9455169.

Chapter 10

Studies:

Fielding, J.W., Fagg, S.L., Jones, B.G., Ellis, D., Hockey, M.S., Minawa, A., Brookes, V.S., Craven, J.L., Mason, M.C., Timothy, A., Waterhouse, J.A. & Wrigley, P.F. (1983). 'An interim report of a prospective, randomised, controlled study of adjuvant chemotherapy in operable gastric cancer,' British Stomach Cancer Group. *World Journal of Surgery*, 7(3), 390–399. https://doi.org/10.1007/BF01658089. PMID: 6349141.

O'Sullivan, P, (Study not yet published as of April 2025)

Linskens, F.G.F., van der Scheer, E.S., Stortenbeker, I., Das, E., Staal, J.B. & van Lankveld, W. (2023). 'Negative language use of the physiotherapist in low back pain education impacts anxiety and illness beliefs: a randomised controlled trial in healthy respondents.' *Patient Education and Counseling*, 110, 107649. https://doi.org/10.1016/j.pec.2023.107649. Epub 27 January 2023. PMID: 36764063.

Chapter 11

Books:

Tolle, E, *The Power of Now*, Yellow Kite, 2001

Hansa, P, *Autobiography of a Yogi*, Self-Realization Fellowship, 2006

Singer, M, *The Untethered Soul*, New Harbinger, 2007

Banks, S, *The Missing Link*, Lone Pine Publishing, 2016

McCammon, J, *Finding Mystery Within*, Julie McCammon, 2021

People:

Deepak Chopra: www.deepakchopra.com

Deborah Epstein: https://deborahepstein.substack.com/p/transform-fear-into-freedom-the-power

Chapter 12

Lectures:

Sydney Banks, Hawaii lecture series: www.sydbanks.com/hawaii

People:

Deborah Epstein: www.deborahepsteinstudio.com

Books:

Pert, C, *Molecules of Emotion*, Simon & Schuster, 1999

Banks, S, *In Quest of the Pearl*, Lone Pine Media, 2021

Chapter 13

Books:

Banks, S, *The Missing Link*, Lone Pine Publishing, 2016

People :

Mooji: mooji.org/mooji and mooji.org/books/an-invitation-to-freedom

Other resources

Banks, S, *The Enlightened Gardener Revisited*, Lone Pine Media, 2005

Banks, S, *Second Chance*, Random House, 1987

Neill, M, *The Inside-Out Revolution*, Hay House, 2013

Neill, M, *The Space Within*, Hay House, 2016

Karn, M, *It's That Simple*, Caffeine for the Soul Press, 2023

Sapolsky, R.M, *Why Zebras Don't Get Ulcers*, S Martin's Press, 2004

Adriaan Louw, *Why Do I Hurt?* International Spine & Pain Institute, 2013

Moseley, L, *Painful Yarns*, Orthopedic Physical Therapy Products, 2007

With Deepest Gratitude

To Linda Sandel Pettit –
Your wisdom landed like stardust on the page.
With grace and patience, you midwifed the words
when I could barely hear them whisper.
In the quiet spaces where doubt lingered,
your voice rang steady –
a lighthouse when I felt lost at sea.
This book carries your fingerprints in the spaces
between what is said and what is felt.

To Dr Bill Pettit –
A kind and steady mirror,
you listened not just to the words,
but to the heart beating beneath them.
With reverence for truth and clarity of mind,

you shepherded this work back to its roots –
to the soul of the Principles,
to the science of healing,
to the simplicity of love.
Your generosity is woven into these pages.

To Mark Howard, Ian Watson, Dominic Scaffidi,
Carol Davis, John F. Barnes, Jamie Smart, Ankush Jain
and Ellen Friedman –
You lent your eyes,
your hearts,
your time –
and in doing so, you lent me courage.
Thank you for seeing something worth sharing
in the fragile first draft.
Your encouragement breathed life
into what might have stayed hidden.

To Peter –
My constant, my compass, my home.
While I wandered through forests of thought,
you stood with quiet faith at the edge,
holding the light.
This book was written in the spaces
you made possible.
Your love is the soil in which this grew.

To Clare, Paula, Joanne and Karen –
You were the first to say yes
to something unformed,
to a whisper of an idea, not yet a book.

With Deepest Gratitude

With open hearts and willing spirits,
you stepped into the unknown beside me.
You let me fumble and find my voice.
You trusted me with your stories,
your pain, your hope –
and in witnessing your transformation,
I was transformed.
This book began with you.
It is, in truth,
a love letter born from that first circle of healing.

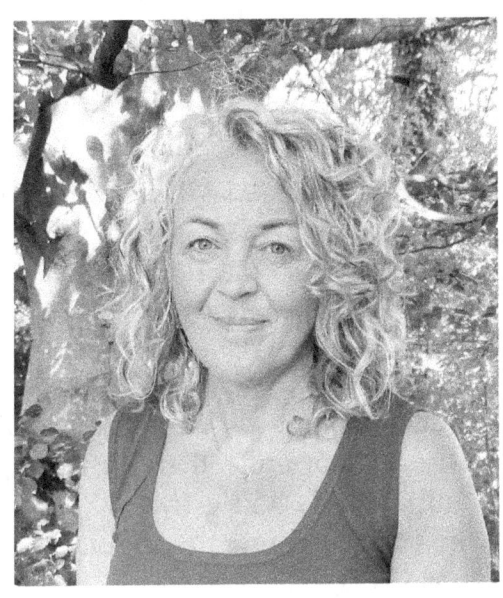

Julie McCammon is a physiotherapist and expert-level practitioner of the John F. Barnes approach to Myofascial Release (MFR). She also works as a Bodymind Coach, having one-to-one conversations with those who struggle with chronic pain or anxious thinking. Currently based in Northern Ireland, she runs her own private practice and holistic healing space, The Garden Room. Here, she assists her clients in their quest to resolve pain and optimise their health. She also helps to guide people with seemingly endless chronic pain and anxiety to freedom through retreats and online offerings.

Her first book, *Finding Mystery Within*, is a self-published memoir that evolved from her 35-year career in healing and the journey she took to rediscover the self-worth she lost as a child. In it, she beautifully blends her unique experiences with an intimate grasp of bodywork and invites us to transform our pain into passion.

Her second book, *Quiet Mind Quiet Body*, combines the latest in pain neuroscience with a psychospiritual understanding called the Three Principles. It bridges the gap between science and spirituality, offering hope to those struggling with persistent pain.

Julie is a wife and mother of two adult children. She continues to support them and others in their pursuits of self-discovery, authenticity, and growth. You can find out more at her website, www.quietmindquietbody.co.uk, or email her at julie@mfrni.com

www.ingramcontent.com/pod-product-compliance
Lightning Source LLC
Chambersburg PA
CBHW050328010526
44119CB00050B/723